Emergency Triage

Second Edition

Emergency Triage

Manchester Triage Group

Second Edition

EDITED BY

Kevin Mackway-Jones
Janet Marsden
Jill Windle

Blackwell
Publishing

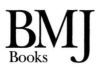

© 2006 by Blackwell Publishing Ltd
BMJ Books is an imprint of the BMJ Publishing Group Limited, used under licence

Blackwell Publishing Inc., 350 Main Street, Malden, Massachusetts 02148-5020, USA
Blackwell Publishing Ltd, 9600 Garsington Road, Oxford OX4 2DQ, UK
Blackwell Publishing Asia Pty Ltd, 550 Swanston Street, Carlton, Victoria 3053, Australia

First published 1996
Second edition published 2006

2   2006

Library of Congress Cataloging-in-Publication Data

Emergency triage / Manchester Triage Group ; edited by Kevin Mackway-Jones, Janet
Marsden, Jill Windle.– 2nd ed.
   p. ; cm.
  ISBN-13: 978-0-7279-1542-9 (pbk.)
  ISBN-10: 0-7279-1542-8 (pbk.)
   1. Triage (Medicine)—Great Britain.   2. Hospitals–Emergency service—Great Britain.
3. Emergency nursing—Great Britain.
   [DNLM: 1. Triage–methods.   2. Emergency Service, Hospital. WX 215 E562 2005]
I. Mackway-Jones, Kevin.   II. Marsden, Janet.   III. Windle, Jill.   IV. Manchester Triage
Group.

  RA975.5.E5E56 2005
    362.18–dc22

ISBN-13: 978-0-727915-42-9
ISBN-10: 0-727915-42-8

A catalogue record for this title is available from the British Library

Set in 9.5/12pt Meridien & Frutiger by TechBooks, New Delhi, India
Printed and bound in Harayana, India by Replika Press Pvt Ltd

Commissioning Editor: Mary Banks
Development Editor: Veronica Pock
Production Controller: Debbie Wyer

For further information on Blackwell Publishing, visit our website:
www.blackwellpublishing.com

The publisher's policy is to use permanent paper from mills that operate a sustainable
forestry policy, and which has been manufactured from pulp processed using acid-free
and elementary chlorine-free practices. Furthermore, the publisher ensures that the text
paper and cover board used have met acceptable environmental accreditation standards.

Contents

Editors

Kevin Mackway-Jones, FAEM Professor of Emergency Medicine, Consultant Emergency Physician, Manchester Royal Infirmary, Medical Director, Greater Manchester Ambulance Service, Honorary Civilian Consultant Advisor in Emergency Medicine, British Army.

Janet Marsden, Senior Lecturer in Healthcare Studies, Manchester Metropolitan University, Nurse Practitioner, Manchester Royal Eye Hospital, Manchester, Chair Ophthalmic Nursing Forum, Royal College of Nursing.

Jill Windle, Lecturer Practitioner in Emergency Nursing, Hope Hospital Salford and University of Salford, Chair, Faculty of Emergency Nursing, Royal College of Nursing.

Members of the original Manchester Triage Group

Kassim Ali, Consultant in Emergency Medicine

Simon Brown, Senior Emergency Nurse

Helen Fiveash, Senior Emergency Nurse

Julie Flaherty, Senior Paediatric Emergency Nurse

Stephanie Gibson, Senior Emergency Nurse

Chris Lloyd, Senior Emergency Nurse

Kevin Mackway-Jones, Consultant in Emergency Medicine

Sue McLaughlin, Senior Paediatric Emergency Nurse

Janet Marsden, Senior Ophthalmic Emergency Nurse

Rosemary Morton, Consultant in Emergency Medicine

Karen Orry, Senior Emergency Nurse

Barbara Phillips, Consultant in Paediatric Emergency Medicine

Phil Randall, Consultant in Emergency Medicine

Joanne Royle, Senior Emergency Nurse

Brendan Ryan, Consultant in Emergency Medicine

Ian Sammy, Consultant in Emergency Medicine

Steve Southworth, Consultant in Emergency Medicine

Debbie Stevenson, Senior Emergency Nurse

Claire Summers, Consultant in Emergency Medicine

Jill Windle, Lecturer and Practitioner in Emergency Nursing

International Reference Group

Paulo Freitas, Consultant Internal Medicine, Hospital Fernando Fonseca, Lisbon, Portugal

Antonio Marques, Consultant Anaesthesiologist, Hospital Geral de Santo Antonio, Oporto, Portugal

Rui Vieira, Nurse Co-ordinator of the Emergency Department, Hospital Fernando Fonseca, Lisbon, Portugal

David Teixeira, Nurse Sergeant Portugese Navy, Hospital Fernando Fonseca, Lisbon, Portugal

Per Örtenwall, Director ALSG Sweden, Gothenburg, Sweden

Nina Widfeldt, Anaesthetist and Intensivist, Beredskapslakare, PKMC, Sweden

Piet Machielse RN, Teamleader, Accident and Emergency Department, Erarmus Medical Centre, University Hospital Rotterdam, Netherlands

Ronald de Caluwe RN, Teamleader, Accident and Emergency Department, Deventer Hospital, Deventer, Netherlands

Isasia Muñoz, Emergency Co-ordination, Hospital Universitario de la Princessa, Madrid, Spain

Manuel A Blanco-Ramos, General Practitioner, Research Unit, Complexo Hospitalario de Ourense, Spain

Franscisco J Fernandez Lopez, Manchester Product Manager, Innova Auria SL, San Ciprián de Viñas, 32900, Ourense, Spain

Joerg Krey, Project Manager and Senior Nurse, LBK Hamburg – Institut fuer Notfallmedizin, Hamburg, Germany

Heinzpeter Moecke, Medical Director, LBK Hamburg – Klinikum Nord, Hamburg, Germany

Preface to the second edition

It is now over 10 years since a group of senior emergency physicians and emergency nurses first met to consider solutions to the muddle that was triage in Manchester, UK. Little did we realise that the solution to our local problem would be robust enough (and timely enough) to become the triage solution for the whole United Kingdom. Never in our wildest dreams did we imagine that the Manchester Triage System would be generic enough to be adopted around the world. Much to our surprise, however, both of these fantasies are reality, and the MTS is used in many languages to triage tens of millions of Emergency Department attenders each year.

While the basic principles that drive the MTS (recognition of the presentation and reductive discriminator identification) are unchanged, it has become necessary to make some adjustments. The second edition incorporates the outcome of consideration of all the comments passed to us by users over the years (for which we are very grateful). It also seeks to include changes that reflect new practice such as the possibility of revascularisation for patients with stroke. Major changes include, by popular demand, new charts for Allergy and Palpitations together with amalgamations and expansions of other charts to keep the core number at 50. A few new discriminators have been introduced such as *acute neurological deficit* and *significant respiratory history*, while others have been redefined. In particular the discriminator for pain at priority 4 has been changed to *recent pain* to reflect the outcome of research that indicated that this would improve the clinical utility of the system. Overall, however, the changes (while significant) are few.

This new edition also seeks to put triage in the context of changes that are happening in many emergency care systems around the world. In the past 10 years the provision of emergency care has become the focus of political and thereby management attention. In particular the care of those patients with less urgent conditions (who make up the majority in most settings) has become a source of concern, since under-resourced systems that focussed (rightly) on patients with the highest clinical priority inevitably resulted in delayed care for those at the other end of the priority scale. In the consumer age this delay is unacceptable. It was easier to blame the clinical prioritisation system (triage) for this delay than it was to accept that the system was under-resourced, and this has meant that triage became out of vogue in some areas. Our standpoint has always been that triage is vital in all systems or circumstances where demand for care outstrips the ability to deliver it. We continue to believe that these circumstances occur occasionally in even the best managed and resourced systems, and frequently in those with the usual demands and staffing. Thus clinical prioritisation (whether called triage, initial assessment or anything else) remains a central plank of clinical risk management in emergency care, and abandoning it completely is not an option. As we show in one of our new chapters, the outcome of the MTS triage process can be used constructively 'beyond prioritisation' and this underlines its developing usefulness to Emergency Departments.

Kevin Mackway-Jones, Janet Marsden, Jill Windle
Manchester, 2005

Preface to the first edition

Every day, emergency departments are faced with a large number of patients suffering from a wide range of problems. The workload varies from day to day and from hour to hour and depends on the number of patients attending and what is wrong with them. It is absolutely essential that there is a system in place to ensure that these patients are seen in order of clinical need rather than in order of attendance.

In the past year great steps have been made towards establishing a National Triage Scale in the United Kingdom; this follows on from similar work in Australia and Canada. This book is intended to allow practitioners of triage to work to a set standard when applying national scales to the patients presenting to their departments. The members of the mult-professional consensus group that designed this methodology hope that individual practitioners will use it to inform the triage process and ensure that their decisions are both valid and reproducible.

This manual contains the basic knowledge necessary for triage practitioners to begin to build their competence in performing triage. It is hoped that practitioners will find a useful source reference and *aide-memoire*.

Kevin Mackway-Jones, 1996

CHAPTER 1
Introduction

Introduction

Triage is a system of clinical risk management employed in Emergency Departments worldwide to manage patient flow safely when clinical need exceeds capacity. Systems are intended to ensure care is defined according to patient need and in a timely manner. Early Emergency Department triage was intuitive rather than methodological and was therefore neither reproducible between practitioners nor auditable.

The Manchester Triage Group was set up in November 1994 with the aim of establishing consensus amongst senior emergency physicians and emergency nurses about triage standards. It soon became apparent that the Group's aims could be set out under five headings.

> **Development of the common nomenclature**
>
> - Development of common definitions
> - Development of a robust triage methodology
> - Development of a training package
> - Development of an audit guide for triage

Nomenclature and definitions

A review of the triage nomenclature and definitions that were in use at the time revealed considerable differences. A representative sample of these is summarised below.

Red	0	A	0	Immediate	0	1	0
Amber	<15	B	<10	Urgent	5–10	2	<10
		C	<60	Semi-urgent	30–60		
Green	<120	D	<120				
Blue	<240	E	–	Delay acceptable	–	3	–
		FGHI					

Despite this enormous variation it was also apparent that there were a number of common themes running through the different triage systems, and these are highlighted below.

1	0	0	0	0
2	<15	<10	5–10	<10
3		<60	30–60	
4	120	<120		
5	<240	–	–	–

Once the common themes of triage had been highlighted it became possible to quickly agree on a new common nomenclature and definition system. Each of the new categories was given a number, a colour and a name and was defined in terms of ideal maximum time to first contact the treating clinician. At meetings between representatives of Emergency Nursing and Emergency Medicine nationally this work informed the derivation of the United Kingdom triage scale shown below.

Number	Name	Colour	Max time (minutes)
1	Immediate	Red	0
2	Very urgent	Orange	10
3	Urgent	Yellow	60
4	Standard	Green	120
5	Non-urgent	Blue	240

As practice has developed over the past 10 years five-part triage scales have been established around the world. The target times themselves are locally set, being influenced by politics as much as medicine particularly at lower priorities, but the concept of varying clinical priority remains current.

Triage methodology

In general terms a triage method can try and provide the practitioner with the diagnosis, with the disposal, or with a clinical priority. The Triage Group quickly decided that the triage methodology should be designed to allocate a clinical priority. This decision was based on three major tenets – first the aim of the triage encounter in an Emergency Department is to aid both clinical management of the individual patient and departmental management; this is best achieved by accurate allocation of a clinical priority. Second the length of the triage encounter is such that any attempts to accurately diagnose a patient are doomed to fail. Finally it is apparent that diagnosis is not accurately linked to clinical priority, the latter reflects a number of aspects of the particular patient's presentation as well as the diagnosis; for example patients with a final diagnosis of ankle sprain may present with severe, moderate or no pain, and their clinical priority must reflect this.

In outline the triage method put forward in this book requires practitioners to select from a range of presentations, and then to seek a limited number of signs and symptoms at each level of clinical priority. The signs and symptoms that discriminate between the clinical priorities are termed *discriminators* and they are set out in the form of flow charts for each presentation – the *presentational flow charts*. Discriminators that indicate higher levels of priority are sought first, and to a large degree patients who are allocated to the standard clinical priority are selected by default.

The decision making process is discussed in chapter 2, and the triage method itself is explained in detail in chapter 3.

Priority and management

It is easy to become confused between the clinical priority and the clinical management of a patient. The former requires that enough information is gathered to enable the patient to be placed into one of the five defined categories as discussed above; the latter may well require a much deeper understanding of the patient's needs, and may be affected by a large number of extraneous factors such as time of day, the state of the staffing and the number of beds available. Furthermore the availability of services for particular patients will fundamentally affect individual patient flow. Separately staffed "streams" of care for particular patient groups will run at different rates. This does not affect underlying clinical priority which affects the order of care within rather than between streams in such a system. These issues are discussed in more detail in chapter 5.

Training for triage

This book and the accompanying course are attempts to provide the training necessary to allow introduction of a standard triage method. It is not envisaged that reading the book and attending a course can produce instant expertise in triage. Rather this process will introduce the method and allow practitioners to develop competence at using the material available. This is the first step towards competence in using the system and must be followed up by audit and evaluation of the system in use.

Triage audit

The Triage Group spent considerable time trying to pin down 'sentinel diagnoses' – that is diagnoses that could be identified retrospectively and which could be used as markers of accurate triage. For the reasons outlined above it soon became apparent that even retrospective diagnosis could not accurately predict actual clinical priority at presentation.

Successful introduction of a robust audit method is essential to the future of any standard methodology, since reproducibility between individual practitioners and departments must be shown to exist. This is discussed in more detail in chapter 6.

Beyond triage in the emergency department

The concept of triage (determining clinical need as a method of managing clinical risk) and the process outlined in this book (presentational recognition followed by reductive discriminator seeking) is applicable in other settings. In some of these (for example medical, surgical or paediatric assessment units) the system can be implemented in exactly the same way as it is in the Emergency Department. In other settings (for instance primary care, out of hours units) many contacts may be made by telephone. A modification of the MTS can be used and this is outlined in chapter 7.

The information gained during the triage process can also be used in other ways to improve patient care. It is important, for instance, that clinicians recognise any change in the patients' status as early as possible. Early Warning Scores have been applied in many settings to formalise this function. In the Emergency Department the A B C D E discriminators from the MTS can be used in exactly this way, and the 'Manchester Monitor' outlined in chapter 7 is an intuitive way for triage practitioners to put into practice the original exhortation for dynamic triage and that 'every intervention is a triage intervention'.

Finally some users of the MTS may have realised that the outcome of the presentation selection – priority assignment process in MTS is to place individual patients into one of 250 slots in a 50×5 presentation – priority matrix. This 'pigeon-holing' can be used to drive pathways of care in systems that have taken to 'streaming'. Particular presentations – priority combinations (e.g. wounds – green, chest pain – orange) may be appropriate to particular streams (minor injuries and resuscitation respectively in the examples given). This concept is discussed in more detail in chapter 8, and an example streaming disposal is now given on each chart.

Summary

Triage is a fundamental part of clinical risk management in all departments when clinical load exceeds clinical availability. Emergency Triage promulgates a system that delivers a teachable, auditable method of assigning clinical priority in emergency settings. It is not designed to judge whether patients are appropriately in the emergency setting, but to ensure that those who need care receive it appropriately quickly. It can be used to monitor care and to signpost streams of care – these will be determined by local provision and actual availability.

CHAPTER 2

The decision-making process and triage

Introduction

Decision making is an essential and integral part of medical and nursing practice. Sound clinical judgement about patient care requires both thought and intuition, and both of these must be based on professional knowledge and skill. Many practitioners argue that critical decision making is only about 'common sense' and 'problem solving', and to a certain extent they are correct. It is, however, more than this and requires a certain level of skill. Within the decision making process clinicians are expected to

> Interpret
> Discriminate
> Evaluate

the information they gather about patients, and critically appraise their actions following that decision. Without a framework of reference on which to base these decisions, they will be unstructured, haphazard and potentially unsafe. The ability to make sound decisions is essential for good patient care.

Triage has been a nursing function for sometime now. For over a decade in the 1980s the only common approach adopted was Blythin's SOAPE assessment tool. That structured the interview but gave no guidance about the outcome. Thus the *outcome* of the triage process was not based on a sound methodology – triage decisions made about patients were potentially unique to each nurse and inherently part of their own decision making process. Such decisions may be fundamentally flawed without a framework of reference. This problem can only be overcome by providing this framework of reference (methodology) for the process of triage, and by designing a method by which practitioners can obtain the necessary skills needed for its implementation.

The development of expertise

A relationship between experience and skill acquisition has been described in which there are five stages of development shown below.

Novice
Advanced beginner
Competent
Proficient
Expert

As practitioners develop along this continuum they acquire skills and learn from their experiences in practice. Overall their decision making ability alters and improves. This process can be facilitated by providing a system based upon a common framework that is methodologically sound, on which decisions can be based and their effectiveness evaluated.

Decision-making strategies

A number of strategies are used in the decision-making process. These are shown below.

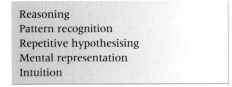

Reasoning
Pattern recognition
Repetitive hypothesising
Mental representation
Intuition

Reasoning

There are essentially two types of reasoning involved in critical thinking: inductive and deductive. Inductive reasoning is the ability to consider all possibilities, and is particularly useful for the less experienced. It involves a time consuming process of considering all patient information collected in order to reach a sound decision about the care they require.

Deductive reasoning is the simultaneous 'weeding out' of possible solutions whilst actively collecting patient information. This strategy is often unknown or unrecognised and becomes part of expert practice. It allows the practitioner to rapidly sort relevant from irrelevant information to reach a decision.

Pattern recognition

This is the strategy most commonly used by clinicians, and is particularly important when making rapid decisions based on limited information that are necessary during triage. Pattern recognition is a method of piecing information together in an analytical sense. Clinicians interpret the pattern of the patient signs and symptoms by comparison with relationships and conditions from previous cases. This leads them to a diagnosis or decision about the patients well-being. The ability to utilise this decision-making skill develops with experience, and often appears to be intuition. Novice, proficient or merely competent practitioners may need to use conscious problem solving to reach a solution, while their more experienced colleagues can employ pattern recognition.

Repetitive hypothesising

Repetitive hypothesising is used by clinicians to test diagnostic reasoning. By gathering data to confirm or eliminate a hypothesis, a decision can be made. Depending on the level of expertise this method can be either inductive or deductive.

Mental representation

Mental representation is a method of simplifying the situation to provide a general picture, and allow focussing on relevant information. This strategy is often used when a problem is very complex or overwhelming. The use of analogies helps the clinician visualise the situation by simplifying the problem and allowing a different perspective. Triage decisions need to be rapid and this method has limited use at this stage in the patients care.

Intuition

Intuition is inextricably linked with expertise, and is commonly seen as the ability of practitioners to solve problems with relatively little data. Intuition rarely involves conscious analysis and is often expressed as 'gut feeling' or 'strong hunch'. Expert practitioners view situations holistically and draw on past experience. Much of their knowledge is embedded in practice and referred to as tacit, where effective decisions are made by combining knowledge with decision making theories and intuitive thought. Many expert nurses are not aware of the mental processes they employ in the assessment and management of patients. Although intuition has remained unmeasurable, the value to clinical practice is acknowledged and well documented.

Decision making during triage

Despite all the theories, decision making is quite simply a series of steps to reach a conclusion and consists of three main phases: identification of a problem, determination of the alternatives and selection of the most appropriate alternative. An approach to making critical decisions has been described which uses the following five steps.

- Identify the problem
- Gather and analyse information related to the solution
- Evaluate all the alternatives and select one for implementation
- Implement the selected alternative
- Monitor the implementation and evaluate outcomes

This approach incorporates a number of theories and methods. When applied to triage the decisions are formed as follows.

Identify the problem

This is done by obtaining information from the patients, their carers and/or any pre-hospital care personnel. This phase allows the relevant presentational flow diagram to be identified.

Gather and analyse information related to the solution

Once a flow diagram has been identified this phase is facilitated since discriminators can be sought at each level. The flow diagrams facilitate rapid assessment by suggesting structured questions. Pattern recognition also plays a part at this stage.

Evaluate all alternatives and select one for implementation

Clinicians collect massive amount of data about the patients they deal with. These are collated into their own mental database and stored in compartments for easy recall; it is most effective when linked to an assessment or organisational framework. These frameworks serve as guides for assessment and are organised as compartments with sub-headings. The presentational flow diagrams provide the organisational framework to order the thought process during triage. Flow diagrams have been found to link the decision-making process into the clinical setting. They aid decision making by providing a structure, and also support junior staff as they acquire decision-making skills.

Implement the selected alternative

There are only five possible triage categories to select from and, as discussed in chapter 1, these have specific names and definitions. Triage practitioners apply the category depending upon the urgency of the patient's condition. Once the priority is allocated the appropriate pathway of care begins.

Monitor the implementation and evaluate outcomes

Triage is dynamic and must be responsive to both patient and departmental needs. The method of triage outlined in this book ensures that the process of reaching the decision is as set. Nurses will therefore be able to identify how and why they reached the outcome (category). This facilitates reassessment and subsequent confirmation or change in the category for instance by using the Manchester Monitor. As important as this is the fact that the whole process can be audited and fed back into the system.

Changing current decision-making practice

For many experienced nurses the introduction of a new framework for triage decisions poses some problems. It is difficult to unlearn individual methods of decision making which have developed over years of practice. However this change should be viewed as a further refinement of their present system, providing for the first time a clear rationale for their decisions and an auditable system. This systematic approach will be a major contribution to the body of knowledge when used to teach junior staff, who rely so heavily on experts to inform and guide their own practice. The actual process of triage decision making presented in this manual is effective and adaptable to any practice setting, and has value to nurses irrespective of their level of experience.

CHAPTER 3
The triage method

Introduction

The method which is outlined in this book has been designed to allow the Triage Practitioner to rapidly assign a clinical priority to each patient. The system selects patients with the highest priority first and works without making any assumptions about diagnosis; this is deliberate and recognises that Emergency Departments are to a large extent driven by the patients presenting signs and symptoms. As discussed in chapter 2 the decisions surrounding triage follow five steps:

- Identify the problem
- Gather and analyse information related to the solution
- Evaluate all the alternatives and select one for implementation
- Implement the selected alternative
- Monitor the implementation and evaluate outcomes

Identifying the problem

Clinical practice is geared around the concept of *presenting complaint* – that is the chief sign or symptom identified by the patient or carer. A list of presentations pertinent to triage is shown below.

Abdominal pain in adults	Behaving strangely
Abdominal pain in children	Bites and stings
Abscesses and local infections	Burns and scalds
Allergy	Chest pain
Apparently drunk	Collapsed adult
Assault	Crying baby
Asthma	Dental problems
Back pain	Diabetes

Continued

Diarrhoea and vomiting	Overdose and poisoning
Ear problems	Palpitations
Exposure to chemicals	Pregnancy
Eye problems	PV bleeding
Facial problems	Rashes
Falls	Self-harm
Fits	Sexually acquired infection
Foreign body	Shortness of breath in adults
GI bleeding	Shortness of breath in children
Headache	Sore throat
Head injury	Testicular pain
Irritable child	Torso injury
Limb problems	Unwell adult
Limping child	Unwell child
Major trauma	Urinary problems
Mental illness	Worried parent
Neck pain	Wounds

This list was reached after considerable discussion and covers almost all presentations to Emergency Departments. It has been refined slightly in this edition to include new charts on allergy and palpitations while the nasal problem chart has been expanded into facial problems, diarrhoea and vomiting have been amalgamated and haematological disease has been incorporated into the general medical charts. The presentations fall broadly into the categories of illness, injury, children, abnormal and unusual behaviour, and major incidents.

The first part of the triage method requires the practitioner to select an appropriate presentation from the list. By selecting the appropriate presentation the practitioner is led to a *presentational flow chart*; the chart identifies discriminators which allow the clinical priority to be determined.

Great care has been taken to ensure that the charts are consistent in their approach, since it is recognised that a number of patients' chief complaints may lead to more than one presentational flow chart. Thus a patient who is feeling unwell with a stiff neck and a headache will be given the same priority whether the practitioner uses the *Unwell Adult, Neck Pain* or *Headache* flow charts.

The charts themselves are shown later in the book.

Gathering and analysing information

To a large degree the patients' presentation will dictate which presentational flow diagram is selected. Following this selection, information must be gathered and analysed to allow the actual priority to be determined. The flow diagram structures this process by showing key discriminators at each level of priority – the assessment is carried out by finding the highest level at which the answer posed by the discriminator question is positive. Discriminators are deliberately posed as questions to facilitate the process.

Discriminators

Discriminators, as their name implies, are factors that discriminate between patients such that they allow them to be allocated to one of the five clinical priorities. They can be *general* or *specific*. The former apply to all patients irrespective of their presentation and therefore appear time and time again throughout the charts; on each occasion the general discriminators will lead the Triage Practitioner to allocate the same clinical priority. Specific discriminators are applicable to individual presentations or to small groups of presentations, and tend to relate to key features of particular conditions. Thus while *severe pain* is a general discriminator, *cardiac pain* and *pleuritic pain* are specific discriminators. General discriminators appear in many more charts than specific ones. All the discriminators used are defined in the discriminator dictionary at the end of the book, and the definitions of the specific ones in use on individual charts are repeated on the accompanying chart notes for ease of reference. All the specific discriminators have been reviewed for the present edition. Key additions include *acute neurological deficit* and *significant respiratory history* which are designed to ensure that patients with stroke and unstable COPD respectively receive early assessment and investigation.

General discriminators are a recurring feature of the charts, and a proper understanding of them is essential to an understanding of the triage method. Six general discriminators are discussed further here – these are shown in the box.

> Life threat
> Haemorrhage
> Pain
> Conscious level
> Temperature
> Acuteness

Life threat

To a practising Emergency Nurse or Emergency Physician *life threat* is perhaps the most obvious general discriminator of all. Broadly speaking this recognises that any cessation or threat to the vital (ABC) functions places the patient in the first priority group.

Patients who are unable to maintain their own airway for any length of time have an insecure airway. Additionally patients with stridor have significant airway threat – this may be an inspiratory or expiratory noise, or both. Stridor is heard best on breathing with the mouth open. Absence of breathing is defined as no respiration or respiratory effort as assessed by looking, listening and feeling for 10 seconds. Inadequacy is a more difficult concept – but in general patients who are failing to breathe well enough to maintain adequate oxygenation have inadequate breathing. There may be an increased work of breathing, signs of inadequate breathing or exhaustion. Absence of pulses is only diagnosed after palpation over a central pulse for 5 seconds. Shock can be difficult to diagnose – the classical signs include sweating, pallor, tachycardia, hypotension and reduced conscious level.

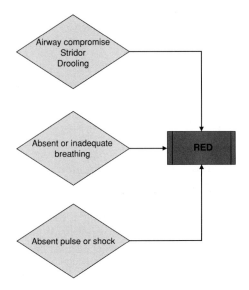

Pain

From the patients' perspective pain is a major factor in determining priority. The use of pain as a general discriminator throughout the presentational flow charts recognises this fact and implies that every triage assessment should include an assessment of pain. Pain assessment is dealt with in detail in chapter 4 and readers are referred there for detailed discussion; in general terms the discriminator severe pain is intended to imply pain that is unbearable, often described as the worst ever, while moderate pain refers to pain that is bearable but intense. Any patient with any lesser degree of recent pain should, if no other discriminators suggest a higher categorisation, be allocated the standard rather than the non-urgent priority.

The general pain discriminator describes the intensity or severity of pain only. Other characteristics of pain, such as site, radiation and periodicity, may feature as specific discriminators in particular presentational flow charts.

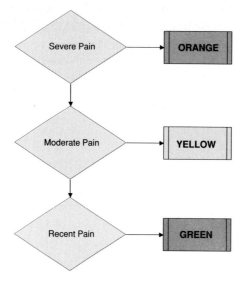

Haemorrhage

Haemorrhage is a feature of many presentations – particularly, but not exclusively, those involving trauma. The haemorrhage discriminators are exsanguinating, uncontrolled major or uncontrolled minor. The use of the success of attempts to control the haemorrhage is deliberate since, in general, continuing bleeding has a higher clinical priority. While of course in practice it can be difficult to decide which category a particular haemorrhage falls into, the definitions of the discriminators are designed to help the practitioner do this. Exsanguinating haemorrhage is present if death will ensue rapidly

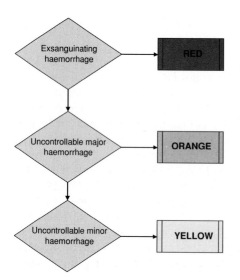

unless bleeding is stopped. A haemorrhage that is not rapidly controlled by the application of sustained direct pressure, and in which blood continues to flow heavily or soak through large dressings quickly is described as an uncontrolled major haemorrhage, while that in which blood continues to flow slightly or ooze is described as uncontrolled minor haemorrhage.

Any bleeding, however moderate, will, unless another discriminator leads to allocation of a higher clinical priority, be allocated to the standard priority.

Conscious level

Conscious level is considered separately in adults and children. In adults only currently fitting patients are always categorised as immediate, whilst all unresponsive children are placed in this clinical priority. Adult patients with altered conscious level (responding to voice or pain or unresponsive) are categorised as very urgent as are children who respond to voice or pain only. All patients with a history of unconsciousness should be allocated to the urgent category.

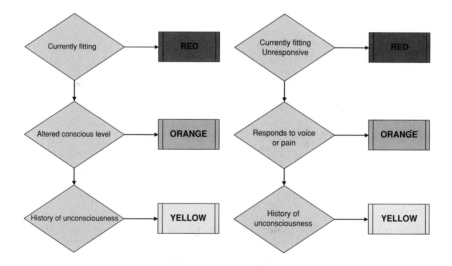

The fact that all patients with alterations in conscious level are allocated to the very urgent priority may be at odds with current practice; this is especially so with regard to the clinical priority given to patients who are intoxicated or under the influence of drugs. Two points need to be made about this: first the aetiology of alterations in level of consciousness is largely irrelevant in determining the risk to the patient – an altered conscious level due to drugs or alcohol is clinically as important as altered conscious level due to other causes. Secondly most drunk patients do not have an altered level of consciousness. Specific points about the allocation of clinical priority to patients who are apparently drunk are dealt with in the presentational flow chart of that name.

Temperature

Temperature is used as a general discriminator. It may be difficult to obtain an accurate measurement during the triage process, although rapid reading tympanic membrane thermometers make this more attainable; clinical impression of skin temperature followed as soon as possible by an accurate assessment of core temperature is an alternative approach.

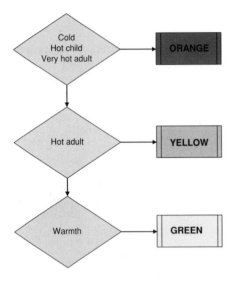

If the skin feels very hot the patient is clinically said to be very hot – this corresponds to a temperature >41°C; similarly if the skin feels hot the patient is clinically said to be hot and this corresponds to a temperature >38.5°C. A patient with warm skin fulfils the discriminator of warmth and this goes with a temperature >37.5°C.

Patients with cold skin can be said to be clinically cold – a core temperature of <35°C matches this.

A very hot adult and hot child will always be categorised as very urgent, whilst a hot adult will be categorised as urgent. Patients who are cold (whatever their age) will be allocated to the very urgent priority.

Acuteness

Within this text certain conventions have been used to help with consistency. The term abrupt is used to indicate onset within seconds or minutes, rapid to indicate less than 12 hours and acute to indicate a time period of 12–24 hours. Recent symptoms and signs are those that have appeared within the past 7 days.

Whilst most clinicians have no problem accepting that the acuity of onset can help indicate the clinical priority, it is slightly more controversial to

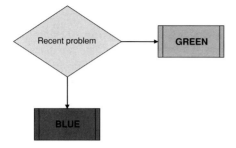

argue that chronicity (in this case greater than 7 days) is used to define a non-urgent problem. However on reflection it is intuitive that the relatively long time that the problem has been present indicates that the patient can be allocated the non-urgent priority (i.e. to wait up to 4 hours) without clinical risk. The triage method is such that the presence of any other general or specific discriminators relevant to the presentation will result in allocation of a higher priority.

The use of this discriminator is not intended to 'punish' patients for turning up 'inappropriately', nor is it intended to ensure that patients who have had injuries or illnesses for a long time have extended waiting times. The actual waiting time for patients with stable problems not of recent onset will depend on the current case mix and case load of the department, and the resources available.

Secondary triage

It may not be possible to carry out all the assessments necessary at the initial triage encounter – this is particularly so if the workload of the department is high. In such circumstances the necessary assessments should still be carried out, but as secondary procedures by a receiving nurse. More time consuming assessments (such as blood glucose estimation and peak flow measurement) are often left to the secondary stage. Many charts have a 'risk limit' placed on them. This indicates the lowest priority that can be applied to the patient if all observations needed are not complete.

Evaluating alternatives and selecting one

Selection of a presentational flow chart leads to the selection of a number of general and specific discriminators which can then be tested against the patient. The skill in implementing the triage method presented here lies in the evaluation of this testing. Practitioners must decide whether the criteria for the presence of certain discriminators are fulfilled, and must decide which of the discriminators that are present lead to the highest clinical priority.

Implementing the selected alternative

This step is essentially a procedural one. The inevitable outcome of the information gathering, analysis and evaluation discussed above will be the decision
that a particular discriminator (general or specific) is the highest positive one.
This leads to allocation of one of the clinical priorities shown in the box.

Number	Name	Colour
1	Immediate	Red
2	Very urgent	Orange
3	Urgent	Yellow
4	Standard	Green
5	Non-urgent	Blue

Documentation

Implementation involves recording the allocated priority. The triage method
outlined here allows documentation to be very simple and precise. All that is
required is a record of which presentation chart is being used, which discriminator defines the category and which category has been selected. Thus, for
instance, the triage record of a patient with chest pain might be as shown in
the box.

Chest pain
Pleuritic pain
Urgent

   This simple approach to documentation not only allows for simple audit but
also means that the reasons for the decision are quite overt.

Patient assessment

The purist view of the triage event is a rapid and focussed encounter in which
information is gathered and applied to assign a priority. This type of assessment
is a skill in itself. The following framework can be used to teach the process to
nurses, ensuring decisions are based on relevant and appropriate patient data.
   It is important that the assessment of a patient is systematic and all elements
of that assessment are pieced together to give a complete picture of the patient's problem. For this reason the triage practitioner should have sufficient
experience of emergency care and the interpersonal skills to communicate
effectively with patients and their families.

The approach to this assessment should take the following format:

Assessment component	Triage activity
Greeting the patient	The assessment begins at first sight of the patients, look at the patients as they approach the triage area, and pick up on any visual signs which may include: • Level of mobility • Obvious injury • Age of patient
The patient history	Ask the patients what has brought them to the emergency department This is a short, concise, subjective history and tells you about the patients' injury/illness/health related problem
The presenting complaint	Patients' presenting complaint can be established from the subjective history they provide *This leads the nurse to choose the most appropriate presentation flow chart*
The focussed questions (interview)	This is where the triage practitioners' knowledge and skills are most evident. Application of anatomical knowledge, pattern recognition of presenting complaints and the ability to react effectively to life threatening situations are all the domain of the triage practitioner Focussed questions can be used to obtain more detail if required e.g. duration of the problem, mechanism of injury, current medications, etc. *The format of these questions will be directed by the discriminators in the chosen presentation flow chart*
Physical examination and assessment of physical parameters	If appropriate: Location of actual sites of injury Recording of baseline observations, pulse, temperature or more detailed information, e.g. obtained from pulse oximetry or assessment of visual acuity
Pain assessment	An integral part of the MTS, both subjective (patient) and objective (triage practitioner) pain scores are worth recording with documentation of rationale for differing scores
Priority/plan of care	Priority assigned using the highest discriminator applicable to the patient Briefly describe any further care identified as a result of the triage assessment

Continued

Assessment component	Triage activity
Documentation	The recording of this information should be to an agreed format and again clear, concise and relevant to the presenting complaint When a computerised triage system is in place the triage practitioner should make sure the focus of attention is always the patient and not the computer screen/keyboard Include a record of any: • Allergies • Current medications • Relevant past medical history • First aid measures applied at triage • Observations • Drugs administered e.g. analgesia **Signature legible**
Reassessment	Document where there is a need to reassess, in particular when analgesia has been administered at triage

By following this systematic process, facilitated by the triage methodology, the patient assessment can be performed rapidly and confidently to reach an appropriate clinical priority in order to guide decision making.

Monitoring and evaluating

Clinical priority can change and triage must therefore be dynamic. The triage method described here can be carried out rapidly and reliably by trained staff; it is therefore useful as a tool for multiple re-evaluations of clinical priority during the patients' stay.

Every nursing encounter can be used as a triage assessment, and any change in clinical priority can be rapidly notified and acted upon. The Manchester Monitor is discussed in Chapter 8.

CHAPTER 4
Pain assessment as part of the triage process

Introduction

Little information is available about the pain experienced by patients present-ing to the Emergency Department, but that that is suggests that pain is a key issue for patients, that staff assess pain poorly and that pain management is suboptimal (oligoanalgesia). Pain is therefore an important issue for a number of reasons.

> - The majority of patients attending Emergency Departments have some degree of pain
> - The amount of pain influences the urgency
> - The adequacy of pain management is a key criterion for patient satisfaction
> - Patients in pain can become agitated and aggressive
> - Patients in pain are a source of distress and stress to both staff and other patients
> - Patients have an expectation that their pain will be dealt with

There are a number of advantages in assessing pain as part of the triage pro-cess. First it ensures that patients' pain is managed at the earliest opportunity – if patients are made comfortable it may be possible to re-categorise them to a lower level of priority; this allows staff to be released to treat patients who need to be seen urgently for other reasons. Patient anxiety is reduced and commu-nication is improved. Without pain assessment the provision of appropriate analgesia at triage is not possible.

The pain assessment process at triage

Pain assessment is an integral part of the Manchester triage methodology pre-sented here. This was a deliberate and explicit recognition of the importance of pain for the reasons discussed above. It is recognised that this resulted in quite a few patients being categorised into a higher priority than was traditionally the case: this was a deliberate attempt to change poor practice.

If a patient's pain is to be assessed formally at triage, and the outcome of that assessment is to help determine the urgency with which that patient is to be seen, then all triage practitioners must be competent in assessing pain, and the pain assessment must be valid and reproducible. It is unrealistic to expect that only the patient's subjective assessment will be taken into consideration during this process. By the same token it is inappropriate that the triage nurses make their own subjective assessment of the patient's pain in isolation.

Pain assessment in the Emergency Department

This can be difficult because patients may be under pressure to say that their pain is severe so as to justify their attendance, and some patients, particularly children, may deny that they have pain to avoid having treatment or being admitted to hospital. Some practitioners' assessment and management of pain may be influenced by 'traditional' pathways of care. For example patients who have fractures are offered immediate analgesia, but patients with abdominal pain may not be offered analgesia until the surgeons have seen them.

There may be concerns that a patient will score pain higher if it is thought that this will result in a quicker treatment.

Pain assessment tools

Many Emergency Departments now use a formal pain assessment tool, but many such tools suffer from the fact that they were developed for use with postoperative and chronically ill patients.

There are three main types of pain assessment tools:

Verbal descriptor scales
Visual analogue scales
Pain behaviour tools

Verbal descriptor scales

These scales consist of a number of word descriptors, usually three or five, which are numerically ranked. The most common descriptors are as follows:

None
Slight
Moderate
Severe
Agonising

and the numerical value increases with the severity of the pain. The verbal descriptor scale is short and relatively easy for the patient to use and has been employed in the Emergency Department environment.

Advantages	Disadvantages
It provides a score which is easy for the nurse to analyse	The use of a single word from a limited list may not reflect the pain that the patient is experiencing
It probably produces reliable data	It is not suitable for patients who do not speak English
It can be modified for use in children	It is the patients' subjective assessment

Visual analogue scales

These scales usually consist of a straight line representing varying levels of pain with verbal anchors at each end.

NO	PAIN AS BAD AS
PAIN	IT COULD BE

Patients can mark anywhere on the line. Verbal descriptors can also be added beneath the line in addition to the word anchors. The line can also be broken down to facilitate scoring for evaluation or comparative purposes.

Advantages	Disadvantages
Easy and fast to use and score	Some patients choose to mark the line near one of the verbal anchors
These scales may be more sensitive than verbal descriptors	Certain patients find VAS too abstract to use in particular those in severe pain, those with lower educational abilities or those with impaired motor coordination. Elderly people have some difficulty in using these scales
If used correctly they are reproducible and reliable	

Pain behaviour tools

These tools have been developed relying on the principle that patients who are in pain exhibit certain behaviours and physiological changes. These tools can measure the following:

Verbal response
Body language
Facial expression
Behavioural changes
Conscious level
Physiological changes

A number of different tools exist, each based on combining a number of the above factors.

Advantages	Disadvantages
Can be used in patients with communication problems	Complex scales. Comparison and scoring are difficult
	The patients' subjective assessment is not included
	Difficult to ensure that pain alone underlies the observed changes
	Time consuming, taking 5–15 minutes to use

The ideal pain assessment tool

An ideal tool for use in the Emergency Department should be simple and quick to use, should have been validated and must give reliable, reproducible results. These results should take account of both patient and observer data.

The pain ruler

No single pain assessment tool is better than another, although some would seem to be more suited to particular clinical areas than others. The pain ruler is a well established pain assessment tool which would seem to lend itself for use in the Emergency Department setting more than some others. In particular the advantages are as follows:

- It measures the intensity of pain and the effects on normal function
- It combines the use of verbal descriptors and a visual analogue scale
- It is fast and easy to use
- It is easily weighted to allow pain assessment, to be part of the triage process
- By helping in the normal function assessment, the nurse can become involved in the pain assessment process
- It promotes dialogue which in turn encourages the patients that their pain is being taken seriously
- It produces a score facilitating ongoing assessment
- The outcome of the assessment is quick and easy to document
- It can easily be adapted for use in children

A pain ruler is shown in the following figure.

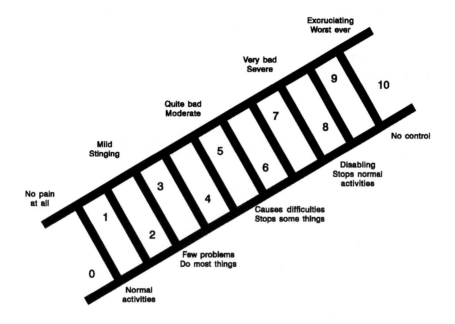

This can be supplemented by a faces scale for use in small children as shown in the following figure.

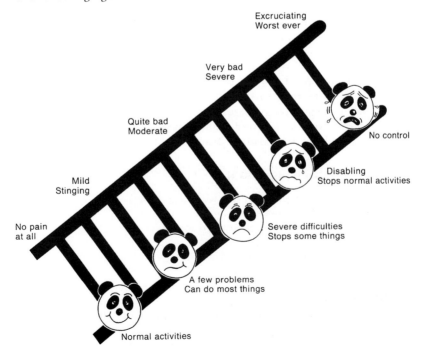

Pain assessment at triage

Pain assessment is a skilled process in any environment and the assessment carried out during triage is no exception. There are particular constraints in this setting reflecting the emergency nature of the patients and the lack of assessment time. Nevertheless, an accurate assessment of the patient's pain into one of the categories shown in the figure is essential if proper and timely care is to be given.

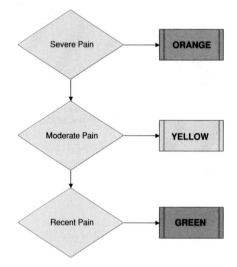

The triage nurse must take into account a number of factors that influence the patients' perception of their pain.

Age

Children may imagine the worst possible outcome of their pain. They use catastrophic thinking which increases their anxiety and fear and may therefore enhance their perception of pain.

Many elderly people suffer from multiple pain problems and may consider a significant pain level to be normal. Many accept pain and cope well with it.

> **Assessment Skill**
>
> • Recognise patients whose age affects pain assessment:
> • Is pain perception increased or decreased?
> • How can this be overcome?

Previous experience of pain

Patients are influenced by their previous experiences of pain. They may compare this pain to previous episodes as to whether this is more or less severe. They will also be influenced by how the pain was managed previously

Assessment Skill

- Recognise whether the patient has had similar pain before
- What is different now?
- How did the patient manage the pain before?

Culture

Illness behaviour, and therefore pain behaviour, has a strong cultural component, and because of different cultural and social influences, not all individuals express pain in the same way. Pain behaviour continues to be reinforced throughout life by the social group to which the individual belongs.

Particular cultural groups do not feel pain less than others, they only differ in how they respond to, or express, their pain. It is essential that the triage nurses recognise that their own cultural and social background will inevitably influence how they interpret a patient's pain behaviour. This identifies one particular difficulty with relying on assessment tools that consider only the patient's (or the nurse's) subjective assessment.

Assessment Skill

- Recognise your own and the patient's cultural background
- How does this affect the patient's pain perception?
- How does this affect the observer's interpretation of behaviour?

Anxiety

There is a link between high anxiety levels and high pain scoring. Patients can be anxious for a number of reasons: they may be concerned about the effect of the illness/accident on their ability to carry out their everyday activities, and they may be anxious about attending hospital or worried about what is actually wrong with them.

There are considerable benefits in addressing a patient's pain at triage, in that the patient is shown at the earliest opportunity that his pain is being taken seriously. Reassurance and explanation from the triage nurse at this time may play a part in effectively reducing the level of pain.

Assessment Skill

- Recognise the level of anxiety of the patient
- What lies behind the patient's anxiety?
- How does this affect the patient's perception of pain?

Disruption to patient's usual activities

Any individual functions at a level which is what he, or she, considers to be normal. Pain can destroy the patient's ability to perform at that level, affecting their physical and emotional well-being, their financial situation and their position within society. Patients' perception of their pain will be influenced to some extent by how the pain will stop them functioning normally. It may not be possible to fully assess the level of disruption to the patient's usual activities, but the nurse may be able to help the patients to focus on the effect of the pain by asking pertinent questions such as does the pain stop their eating/drinking/sleeping/breathing properly?, does the pain stop them walking/sitting, does the pain stop them working/going to school?, etc.

> **Assessment Skill**
>
> - Recognise the degree to which normal daily activities are disrupted
> - How can the degree of disruption be assessed?
> - How does the degree of disruption relate to the patient's perception of pain?

If a patient scores his pain as 10 but then is able to perform all his usual activities, the nurse should consider other factors that may be influencing the patient's assessment of his pain.

Other considerations

Some patients may not be able to participate in the pain assessment process.

They may be confused, have learning difficulties or be too distressed. Likewise, they may not be able to read or understand English. Consider each patient as an individual and think about other tools which you could use instead.

> **Assessment Skill**
>
> - Recognise that no single assessment tool is appropriate for every patient presenting with pain
> - Can this patient participate using this method of assessment?
> - What other methods of pain assessment are more appropriate?

CHAPTER 5
Patient management, triage and the triage nurse

Introduction

There is a difference between absolute clinical priority as defined using the method in this book, and relative priority within and between triage categories. In overview the process of triage as outlined here is quite simple – patients are assigned to a triage category and then managed in order of priority and time of attendance. However there are many other factors apart from clinical priority which may from time to time influence how the patient is handled within the Emergency Department. This chapter outlines these factors and discusses their importance. Clinical priority and the findings that determine it are clearly very important, but failure to recognise other factors can be detrimental to both departmental function and quality of care for individual patients.

Type of patient

There are a number of issues about the nature of individual patients that affect their management in addition to their clinical priority. These are summarised below.

Children

Children may need special management, especially in Emergency Departments without special paediatric facilities. They are always accompanied by someone else (usually a parent but teachers, relatives or social workers may also be present), as well as siblings and friends who, although well, need entertaining. Children have very short attention spans and get bored, frightened and tired very easily. They may get very distressed and agitated because of communication and understanding difficulties, and this makes later handling more difficult.

Children who can be happily entertained by a play leader or in a separate waiting room with play facilities probably do not need any special attention other than frequent reassessment. It is helpful if child friendly food and drink e.g. snacks and drinks in cartons, bottles, etc. are available (provided the carer of any child who may need a general anaesthetic or sedation is aware of the need to keep the child nil by mouth).

It may be worthwhile having a special policy for children who present late in the evening or at night. The child who is very tired may prove impossible to examine and treat, so a relatively early examination may be considered.

Elders
Relative immobility can cause increased discomfort in the waiting room and may cause difficulty in reaching the toilet or going for refreshments. A person who is normally able to cope well in familiar surroundings may become quite confused and disorientated in the Emergency Department even if only slightly injured. The elderly are often set in a routine and become anxious if unable to meet their normal time table. There may be carers at home who have responsibilities who would need to be informed about the elderly patients' attendance. The elderly are very prone to pressure damage to tissues which can develop after only half an hour on a hospital trolley. If they cannot be seen quickly for treatment they need frequent nursing attention. They may have problems with continence which if not anticipated may lead to embarrassment. Memory problems may lead to them providing little information. Practitioners should be aware of these issues and consider the relative needs of this group of patients.

Patients with physical disability or learning difficulties
Apart from the extremes of age, there will be patients who have particular difficulties. These include those with special needs, poor sight, poor hearing, etc. Persons who can cope quite well in the community under controlled circumstances may have great difficulties in the strange environment of the Emergency Department. Communications again become particularly important, and it may be appropriate for such patients to be seen relatively quickly.

Abusive/aggressive patients
There are few things worse than having a full waiting room, with one or more patients (or more often relatives or friends of patients) constantly demanding attention. Although the guiding principle must be that these patients are not given priority just because they shout louder, the distress they cause to others must be taken into consideration. An initial attempt to communicate departmental policy may be followed by a number of actions. The patient may be placed in an individual cubicle to wait in order to minimise the disruption to the waiting room. Alternatively such patients can be seen, treated and discharged rapidly for the benefit of others. If all else fails the patient (or the patients relatives) may be asked to leave, assisted as necessary by security or police.

Patients under the influence of alcohol
These patients are difficult to assess because of the effect of alcohol on conscious level and on pain perception. They need frequent assessment to check

that they are not deteriorating or developing a problem not immediately apparent at triage. Disruptive drunk patients should be treated as outlined above.

The regular
Most departments have a number of patients who are frequent attenders. It is undoubtedly tempting to place these patients in the non-urgent category without proper assessment. Beware, even the regulars develop organic pathology, injure themselves or have a serious complication of their disease. These patients (even those with predominantly social problems) are in fact more likely to develop illnesses or sustain injuries than the general population. Each attendance should be treated as a new visit and proper assessment should be undertaken; this avoids underestimation of possible serious causes for attending.

Patients who re-attend
There are occasions when patients return to the department, usually because their original presenting complaint has not resolved or they have developed a complication. Sometimes the patients' expectations of the natural progress of an injury or illness are unrealistic. The patient may also return having failed to wait for definitive treatment on a prior occasion. The patient should be allocated a triage category according to the symptoms presenting at the time of triage, and not according to the original triage category. Some departments may have policies recommending that such patients are reviewed by a senior doctor if available. It may also be appropriate to offer some of these patients a review clinic appointment for assessment by a senior doctor if the problem does not seem to need immediate treatment.

Clinic patients
Most Emergency Departments hold review clinics. Some services hold clinics in an area away from the department, and although they may see Emergency Department staff these patients would not impinge on the triage nurse role. If the clinic is held within the Emergency Department then it is usual for these patients to have a different priority and/or route through the department. It is important that the triage nurse explains to the new patients that there are clinic patients who may be called out of turn.

Patients referred by other agencies

Many departments allow their facilities to be used by other teams for assessment of the patients. These patients are usually pre-arranged or accepted patients from primary care physicians. They are often patients who are accepted for possible admission and many have a relatively high clinical priority. *These patients must be triaged in the same way as Emergency Department patients.* If the patient is triaged as first priority it would be usual for the Emergency Department team to initiate resuscitation, unless the referral team is in the department. The triage nurse should inform the referral team of the triage category of the patients in order to try and ensure that these patients are treated with a similar degree of urgency as Emergency Department patients. It may also be appropriate for the triage nurse to ask departmental clinical staff to provide analgesia or initiate immediate investigations, in order to smooth the patients' stay in the department.

Some patients may have been brought in by the police (for instance under mental health legislation), by social services or by other professional services. Triage practitioners should be aware of the pressures on staff from other agencies and consider this when deciding on the management of such patients.

Departmental factors

Any department that deals with emergencies may at times be overwhelmed by the influx of patients. Sometimes it only takes one seriously ill patient, or an absent member of staff to produce standstill. Each department needs to develop means of coping with this. An accurate triage assessment is an essential first step in good departmental management.

Both the workload and the staffing of the department will vary according to the time of day. Frequently overnight there is reduced clinical staffing. This may cause increased waiting times and difficulties in the waiting room, particularly if there are patients who are aggressive or under the influence of alcohol. It may be appropriate for the clinician to see a few 'quick' cases before spending a long time with a patient of a higher triage category. Some departments may wish children to be seen more rapidly late at night.

Fast tracking, streaming and matching resources to demand

Streaming is a term used to describe the splitting of patients into different groups who are then seen by staff dedicated to their particular stream. Once within a particular stream the patient is not affected by pressures elsewhere in the system. This is similar to the concept of 'fast-tracking' where particular groups of patients (usually those with relatively minor injuries and illnesses) are identified and seen by dedicated staff to improve the flow. The main difference is that streaming is delivered as a planned intervention rather than as a reactive one.

The Manchester Triage System can be used to facilitate streaming. This is discussed in detail in chapter 8.

The quiet days

Even when the department is quiet it is important to maintain the momentum of work in order to ensure that patients are seen promptly within their triage category, and to stop unnecessary delays.

Role of the triage nurse

The triage nurse's main role is the accurate prioritisation of patients, and this must be the prime objective. The triage nurse needs to become accomplished at rapid assessment – this involves quick decision making and suitable delegation of tasks. Long conversations with patients should be avoided as should exhaustive history taking. Clinical observations such as temperature/pulse, etc. need to be delegated if they are not required to establish priority as they are too time consuming.

In small departments the triage nurse will see all patients coming in the department. In others there may be separate nurses dealing with patients who come walking and on stretchers. The mode of arrival of the patient does not always concur with the seriousness of the illness. (Patients with trivial complaints call the Emergency Services and patients with MI arrive by car.) Therefore there must be close liaison between triage staff in order to place the patients correctly. The triage method outlined in this book should assist this process by standardising triage practice.

Rapid influxes of patients may require the triage nurse to seek assistance from another member of staff. The triage process is integral to the clinical management of most departments, and a variety of additional tasks may be undertaken.

First aid/analgesia

The triage nurse may need to provide or facilitate some first-aid treatment, and recognise the need to provide analgesics if required (see pain). Application of a sling or dressing will immediately improve the patient's comfort and help minimise further trauma and bleeding.

Patient information

The triage nurse is the first clinical contact for the patient, and talking the patient through the illness and probable course in the department alleviates much distress and anxiety. Patients appreciate knowing the waiting time, the probable time spent in the department, whether any investigations may be ordered and possible treatment. This information can be provided quite quickly for most common conditions.

Health promotion

The triage nurse (if times allows) can usefully act as a health promoter. The patient is quite receptive to health care advice when an adverse event has occurred. If possible brief advice about relevant topics such as locked cabinets, cycle helmets and stopping smoking may be appropriate. It is helpful if patient information leaflets are available.

Disposition of patients around the department

The triage nurse will often have to decide where to place the patients in the department. This will depend on departmental facilities and policies. Patients who are distressed, in pain, bleeding or at extremes of age may be best placed in cubicles away from the general waiting room. Patients who need to be lying down for examination (for example those suffering from knee injuries, back complaints and abdominal pain) should be placed in an area where they can lie down. Ill patients may well walk into the department and may need to be placed in the appropriate area of the department. To achieve this, the triage nurse needs to be continuously aware of the occupancy of the department and the current disposition of patients.

Managing the waiting room

Until they have been seen by a clinician, the patients' main contact is the triage nurse. Further advice may be sought by these patients, and criticisms delivered. The triage nurse needs to keep the occupants of the waiting room informed of the current approximate waiting time. Constant observation and reassessment are necessary in order to spot those patients whose condition is changing. Triage is a dynamic process and the patients often need regular reassessment. This might occur after an intervention e.g. the administration of analgesic, or after an appropriate length of time. Patients may be dropped into a lower category after pain relief or brought forward if they deteriorate. No one can anticipate all problems and it is not a 'failure' of accurate assessment to change the triage category according to further developments in the patients condition, or indeed with further information that may be acquired. The waiting room should be considered to be a clinical area.

CHAPTER 6
Auditing the triage process

Introduction

When the Manchester Triage Group set out its aims at its very first meeting in November 1994, it clearly identified the need for a robust audit methodology. The reasons for this were very simply that the MTS was designed to reduce unwarranted variations in the triage process and this reduction could only be ensured by audit. Audit, in this context at least, is a quality management procedure; since triage is a fundamental cornerstone of clinical risk management, failure to ensure the quality of triage may have serious consequences.

Fortunately the Manchester Triage methodology is eminently auditable. The presentation – discriminator – priority progression (the process) by which individual triage practitioners arrive at their conclusions – is very easy for an auditor to note and easily assessable for accuracy by a trained assessor. Indeed, experience shows that untrained assessors have good agreement while trained assessors strongly agree in their opinions of the triage process.

In addition to the process of triage discussed above, audit can also address other issues such as completeness of notes and adherence with terminology (it is not unusual for harassed triage practitioners to 'invent' a new discriminator if the actual discriminator has slipped their mind).

The aim of this chapter is to describe a robust triage audit method for the Manchester Triage System and also to outline some of the results that have been found in audits around the world.

Audit method

At a basic level, the accuracy of individual triage practitioners underpins the whole quality agenda. Thus the most robust triage audit continuously assesses the practitioners for accuracy (and is linked by reflective practice and, if necessary, additional training to improved performance). The method outlined below is an audit of individual practitioner triage activity and is designed to audit the quality of decision making against the MTS standard, along with standards of record keeping and documentation.

- All triage practitioners are identified.
- All episodes of triage are identified.
- Episodes are all assigned to individual practitioners.
- 2% of episodes per practitioner (minimum of 10 episodes) are randomly selected.

- Episodes are assessed by a senior trained triage practitioner.
- The completeness of episodes is expressed as a simple proportion.
- The accuracy of episodes is expressed as a simple proportion.
- The number of incomplete episodes is fed back to the practitioner.
- The overall accuracy is fed back to the practitioner.
- Any causes of inaccurate triage are fed back to the practitioner.

To ensure consistency of audit, 10% of episodes assessed are performed independently by a second senior practitioner. Any differences are moderated by discussion. Continuous audit can be time consuming but is an excellent means of assessing standards of triage activity and decision making. A monthly audit is advised when MTS is introduced to a clinical area. Even in large departments triaging 100,000 patients each year, the number audited is only 2,000 cases per year or 160 per month. The frequency of audit may be reduced to 3–6 every month thereafter. A typical audit tool might look like the following.

Criteria	Yes	No	Comments
Correct use of presentational flow chart			
Specific discriminators			*(Record as seen on triage record)*
Pain score recorded			
Correct triage category assigned (based on patient presentation and discriminators)			
Triage record legible and signed			
Retriaged where necessary			

The overall approach is summarised in the flow diagram.

As can be seen from the above, two measures of the triage process are obtained: completeness and accuracy. These are defined below.

Completeness

An episode is complete if all the steps necessary to reach the conclusion have been undertaken. As the method is reductive (that is it assumes everybody is priority one, and works its way down from there) this requires that the practitioner excludes all the discriminators in any higher priority. Thus if SaO_2 appears as a discriminator in the chart selected, then the episode would be incomplete if no result was recorded. The most common failure is to fail to record pain score.

Accuracy

An episode is recorded as accurate if both the presentation and discriminator selected are appropriate. It is important to realise that there may be appropriate alternatives (indeed the system is designed to ensure that this can occur); thus

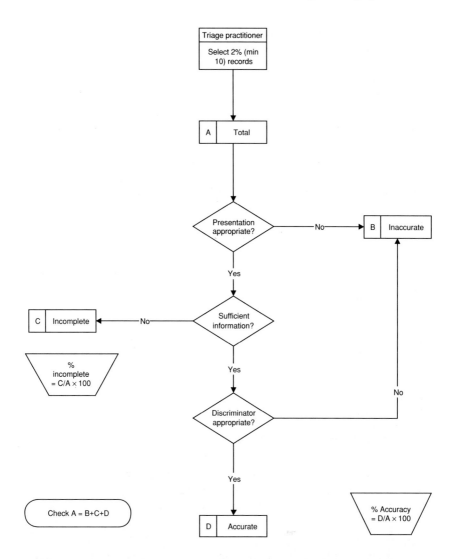

audit should be carried out by a practitioner with sufficient experience to make this judgement.

Targets
- 0% episodes incomplete
- 95% accuracy
- 95% agreement between assessors

Triage in practice

The triage audit will have a number of additional effects on the triage process. It is not possible to carry out the audit without accurate triage notes;

any deficiencies in record making will be highlighted. For instance, failure to record a pain score will mean that the auditor cannot be sure whether the triage priority assignment is correct. This will then be marked as an incomplete episode. Pain scoring will thus be encouraged. Similarly failure to record required physiological measurements such as PEFR in asthma or temperature in the unwell child will result in incomplete episodes. Feedback on a regular basis will improve these assessments. Experience has shown that this is an early 'win' from audit.

Example of a regional audit process

To compare the accuracy of the triage process across a heath region in England, 100 triage episodes from each centre were audited by trained senior triage practitioners. Each card was reviewed by two practitioners and 10% of the cards were triaged independently by a further couple of senior triage practitioners. A strong inter-observer agreement was found.

Accuracy can be seen to vary from 68% to 95%. This allowed informed interpretation of the findings of the audit which demonstrated marked variation in case mix (triage spectrum) across the region. Furthermore a strong association between computerised triage systems and accurate triage was demonstrated.

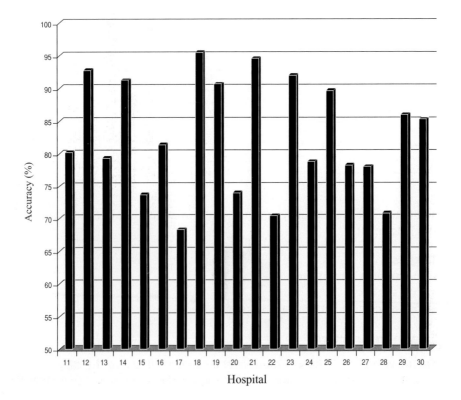

National triage audit

The Manchester Triage System was introduced in Portugal as a national system in 2001 having been trialled in a number of hospitals prior to that time. The system is administered by the Portuguese Triage Group (GPT) that has insisted on audit as an integral part of triage in all its codes of practice. All hospitals implementing MTS are required to audit continuously and report the results of the audit to the GPT at an annual meeting. This audit has shown high overall accuracy.

Interestingly, audit has also demonstrated that the average triage intervention time is between 30 and 60 seconds, which contradicts the assertion that the MTS slows down the Emergency Department process. It would appear that slowing occurs because of tasks other than prioritisation carried out by nurses as part of the initial assessment.

CHAPTER 7
Telephone triage

Introduction

The recognition of the need for formalised telephone triage and its development first occurred in the United States. Telephone triage was first described as a useful tool in the emergency setting in the United Kingdom in 1991. Various benefits have been attributed to this strategy including reduced attendance at the ED due to explanations and self-care advice, redirection of patients to more appropriate agencies, identification of problems before the patient attends the department , cost effectiveness and patient empowerment.

Giving advice by telephone has always been an integral part of the nurse's role although none has been recognised as having a particularly distinct identity. Early studies suggested that patient assessment by telephone was subjective, poorly structured and carried out by untrained personnel. Decisions were made hastily without ascertaining the full facts. Recommendations arising from these studies were that a designated telephone advisor be the first point of contact for telephone advice, protocols for informed advice for common problems should be developed and that adequate documentation was essential. Where these strategies have been implemented in practice, telephone triage has been found to be a safe and effective method of prioritisation. Formalised advice giving by telephone has the potential to be a valuable tool in many settings – a fact that has been recognised in the development of NHS Direct, the telephone advice and help line, in the United Kingdom.

The demarcation line between telephone advice and telephone triage is debatable. It is suggested that triage occurs when a formalised process of decision making takes place which allows identification of clinical priority and allocation to predetermined categories of urgency of need for medical evaluation and care.

Telephone triage methodology

When undertaken effectively, triage involves a decision about clinical priority, which is based on presentation rather than diagnosis. Telephone triage should be undertaken in exactly the same way. The methodology described here builds on the effective face-to-face triage methodology taught by the Manchester Triage Group. The possible outcomes are, however, simplified from the five category system as there are fewer options available to the telephone triage practitioner.

The decisions which must be made are as follows:
- Does the patient need immediate and urgent care? (medicine now)
- Do they need care within the next few hours? (medicine soon)
- Can medical or other care be delayed? (medicine later)

Patients who are in the medicine now category are best served by the Emergency Ambulance Service and Emergency Departments, whatever their locations. Those in the other two categories may have care delivered in a number of locations and by various providers. Thus the time to care in the Medicine Soon category will vary, depending upon the setting in which the telephone triage is located. In ED based triage this might mean that the patients should make their way to the ED as soon as possible. In primary care based triage, the patient might be seen the same day in the nearest available clinic. It is essential that the practitioner undertaking telephone triage is aware of (or has access to information about) current local service organisations such as dental emergency arrangements, telephone numbers of primary care facilities and the location of all night pharmacies.

Making the decision

On receiving the telephone call, the practitioner must gather some basic information from the caller about the nature of the problem. This will dictate which presentational flow chart is selected.

Once the decision has been made, questioning techniques are used to elicit information in order to decide what priority should be allocated.

The methodology is reductive – working from more serious to less serious discriminators, and the nurse is prompted to cover all possibilities by the information contained on the flow charts.

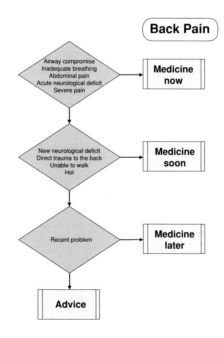

The practitioner must decide whether the criteria for each discriminator are fulfilled, and which of the discriminators present leads to the highest clinical priority. An example chart for back pain is shown above.

Discriminator definitions remain the same when undertaking triage by telephone. The questions normally asked by the triage practitioner must be modified to take into account the remoteness of the patient, the levels of anxiety and the possibility that the caller is not the patient.

Some examples of questions relating to particular discriminators, along with the discriminator definitions, are shown here.

Discriminator	Questions	Definition
Acute onset after injury	Did this start after you fell/were hit, etc.? When did this start?	Onset of symptoms immediately or shortly after a recent physically traumatic event
Acutely avulsed tooth	When did your tooth come out? Was this the result of injury? Is it complete with a root?	A tooth that has been avulsed intact within the previous 24 hours
Acutely short of breath	Have you suddenly become short of breath? Are you more short of breath than normal?	Shortness of breath that comes on suddenly, or a sudden exacerbation of chronic shortness of breath
Altered conscious level	Do they open their eyes or move when you speak to them or gently shake their shoulders?	Not fully alert. Either responding to voice or pain only or unresponsive
Cardiac pain	Where is the pain? Have you had pain like this before? What is it like? Does it go to your arm or neck?	Classically a severe dull 'gripping' or 'heavy' pain in the centre of the chest, radiating to the left arm or to the neck. May be associated with sweating and nausea
Direct trauma to the neck	Have you been hit on your neck? What exactly happened?	This may be top to bottom (loading) for instance when something falls on the head, bending (forwards, backwards or to the side), twisting or distracting such as in hanging
High risk of self-harm	What are you (they) going to do? Do you want to kill yourself?	An initial view of the risk of self-harm can be formed by considering the patients' behaviour. Patients who have a significant history of self-harm are actively trying to harm themselves or who are actively trying to leave with the intent of harming themselves are at high risk

Continued

Discriminator	Questions	Definition
Inconsolable by parent	Can you calm them down at all? Do they settle at all when you cuddle them?	Children whose crying or distress does not respond to attempts by their parents to comfort them fulfil this criteria
Signs of dehydration	Do you (they) have a dry tongue? Do you (they) look dry? Are you (they) passing as much urine as normal?	These include dry tongue, sunken eyes, increased skin turgor and, in small babies, a sunken anterior fontanelle. Usually associated with a low urine output
Signs of meningism	Do you (they) have a stiff neck? Does the light hurt your (their) eyes?	Classically a stiff neck together with headache and photophobia

Interim advice

Because the patient is remote from the nurse, interim advice may be necessary in order to promote recovery or prevent deterioration in the condition of the patient before medical help is accessed. For example if the triage practitioner obtains information that the patient is not breathing properly or has a compromised airway, then lifesaving basic life support advice must be given to the caller so that resuscitation can be taken until help arrives. Similarly if a child is unwell and is triaged to 'medicine later' it may be appropriate to give the carer advice on simple measures to alleviate symptoms such as fever and diarrhoea. Interim advice should be available for each discriminator. Some examples are shown below.

Discriminator	Interim advice
Currently fitting	Attempt to place the patient in a recovery position (describe if necessary). Loosen clothing. Do not attempt to place anything into the mouth
Hot child	Remove warm clothing. Administer Paracetamol elixir if available, dosing according to the manufacturer's recommendations
History of overdose or poisoning	Do not try to induce vomiting. If lips are burning after ingestion of a corrosive substance try frequent sips of cold water
Open fracture	Do not move the limb. Place pads or cushions around it to keep it still. Cover the wound with a clean pad or towel

Once details of the patient's presenting symptoms have been obtained, a priority category allocated and any appropriate interim advice given, then advice on transport may be necessary. Protocols for this will be agreed locally, depending on departmental circumstances.

Pain

Pain assessment is an integral part of the triage decision making process but presents special problems in a telephone triage situation. Not only is observation impossible, but the time taken to elicit specific information about pain may be limited and the patient or carer's understanding of what the triage practitioner means when s/he asks about pain scales may be suboptimal.

The pain evaluation tool within the telephone triage system has been modified to reflect these difficulties. Severe pain is used as a discriminator to prioritise the patient into the 'medicine now' category in all cases. Severe pain warrants urgent investigation and management. Pain does not feature in any other decisions about clinical priority which must be made on the basis of other information gained by the practitioner.

The telephone triage practitioner

Telephone triage, like face-to-face triage, should be undertaken by experienced practitioners. The availability of protocols and charts does not remove the need for expert clinical knowledge. Arguably the decisions made in telephone triage call for a higher level of skill and knowledge than when the patient is present. Furthermore the questioning skills of the practitioner must be very highly developed in order to obtain the most useful information from a troubled caller in the least possible time.

Like face-to-face triage, telephone triage works well when it is carried out correctly and less well when corners are cut, or important aspects such as pain are ignored. Systems must be auditable and this relies on good training of competent practitioners using their skills and knowledge and the tools available to them to the best effect.

The telephone triage methodology provides an effective and auditable tool for the prioritisation of patients presenting to immediate care settings by telephone.

CHAPTER 8
Beyond prioritisation

The Manchester Triage System was designed to be a robust, auditable clinical risk management tool that identified the clinical priority of individual patients. As has been alluded to earlier in this book, the process itself and the outcome of the process can be useful beyond prioritisation. Two such uses are described here.

The Manchester monitor

Triage is a dynamic process and should be undertaken periodically on all patients while they are waiting for treatment. In this way any change in status can be identified and the triage category can be modified if necessary. The need for monitoring does not stop after first clinician contact – it is very important that any later deterioration is identified as soon as possible so that appropriate reassessment can be undertaken and any treatments started. The similarity between post triage monitoring (dynamic triage) and post clinical assessment monitoring is self-evident.

In some areas of the hospital, ongoing monitoring uses an 'early warning score' format very successfully. In the emergency department, however, this requires clinicians to learn and implement a new assessment tool. The discriminators within the MTS, particularly those addressing ABC life threat, lend themselves very well to ongoing assessment. The 'Manchester monitor' adaptation is shown here. The monitor can be used very quickly, using parameters with which ED clinicians are very familiar, to identify deterioration (or improvement) in the patient's condition that might need intervention.

	Red	Orange	Yellow
Airway	Airway compromise		
Breathing	Inadequate breathing	Very low SaO$_2$ Acutely SoB	Low SaO$_2$
Circulation	Shock Exsanguinating haemorrhage	Abnormal pulse Marked tachycardia Uncontrollable major haemorrhage	Uncontrollable minor haemorrhage
Disability	Unresponsive child Hypoglycaemia	Altered conscious level	

As with all monitoring tools, it is change rather than absolute score that is important. Thus the new appearance of a red discriminator should indicate immediate clinical reassessment, while the recognition of an orange or yellow discriminator should precipitate clinical action within 10 or 60 minutes respectively. This approach has the advantage of using a tool with which the nursing staff are familiar within a framework that is also well known.

Presentation-priority matrix mapping

As the idea of the inappropriate patient becomes replaced by the concepts of inappropriate care delivery and patient choice, multiple entry gates to emergency care and the 'emergency care village' become realities. Clinicians must be equipped with tools that enable them to decide safely and effectively where patients might be best managed.

It became clear while reviewing the MTS that the outcome of the prioritisation process could be captured to inform decisions about the most appropriate disposition of the patient. In particular the combination of the presentational chart used and the priority allocated (the presentation-priority complex) could be matched to particular types of provision of emergency care. Thus a patient presenting with a limb problem and allocated to the standard priority should be seen in a minor injury area, while a patient with chest pain allocated to the very urgent priority is best seen in the resuscitation room. The MTS consists of 50 presentations and 5 priorities – making a total of 250 presentation–priority combinations. A mapping exercise was undertaken to consider appropriate disposition of all of these. This disposition matrix using presentation and priority is shown here. The dispositions available will be subject to local emergency care provision. For example, the lack of an emergency eye unit will change where patients with eye problems are managed. It may, however, also stimulate debate with the local ophthalmic service in order to provide a more appropriate service for these patients. The dispositions shown below assume a complete range of emergency care provision, while those shown on the individual charts later in this text assume only basic emergency department and primary care are available.

Black boxes indicate that the MTS does not have the presentation–priority outcome indicated by the box. Where grey boxes appear, it indicates that the disposition may be to two or more services. These are the services appearing in the grey box itself or those on each side of it. The triage practitioner will need to exercise judgement as to which is the most appropriate. This decision will be influenced by the availability of the services, the current pressures on them, the triage discriminator and the patients' choice.

It is apparent that PC and Mi dispositions are professionally led rather than patient led. It would be possible to provide both these services within a single area – perhaps an 'Urgent Care Centre' or 'Rapid Assessment and Treatment Unit'. This approximately maps onto the current 'Minor End' of many Emergency Departments but has obvious potential to coalesce within the Emergency Village with out-of-hours Primary Care provision.

The PA disposition will be provided differently throughout the country and may include psychiatry and psychiatric nursing. Many Emergency Departments have Emergency Psychiatric Nursing Teams and some are developing Psychiatric Assessment Unit functions.

The DC and EC dispositions will depend on local provision. However the decision within grey areas will also depend on opening times and location of any such facilities.

The SHC disposition will again depend on location and opening times of local provision, although the specialist nature of the care delivered will dictate that most patients not requiring immediate or very urgent care are redirected. Experience has shown that triage must be accurate (as assessed by audit) if it is to be used to drive disposition.

Other uses of the triage consultation

Often the triage event includes more than the assessment and prioritisation of patients. In addition to being asked to prioritise patients and deliver basic first aid, practitioners may also be expected to do the following:

- Administer analgesia
- Refer patients directly to have x-ray
- Triage patients to self-care, pharmacy services, GP non-urgent appointments, Out of Hours Service
- Initiate agreed patient pathways to facilitate direct referral to in-patient specialities.

In many cases this will require a higher level of decision making than has previously been expected. There will be some associated training needs in the assessment of patients and understanding of the referral process in order for the nurse to make the choice of service that best meets the patient's needs.

The benefits of 'value added' or extended triage are that patients have access to pain management at the point of access where a delay in definitive treatment may be encountered. There is likely to be a reduction in the of total time spent in the department if patients present to the treating clinician with their x-rays ready for interpretation. Patients may avoid unnecessary delay if directed to alternative services/specialities from triage.

The downside to this approach is that introducing more intervention in the assessment will result in longer consultation times and may create a significant delay for patients entering the system, thus introducing an element of risk. To offset this problem it is feasible to have more than one triage practitioner operating at any given time to ensure all patients are triaged without significant delay. As previously noted the time needed for accurate prioritisation is only 30–60 seconds and it is therefore disingenuous to blame the triage event itself for any delays that result from widening the remit of initial assessment.

	1	2	3	4	5
Abdominal pain in adults	R	R	Ma	PC	PC
Abdominal pain in children	R	R	Ma	PC	PC
Abscesses and local infections	R	R	Ma		PC
Allergy	R	R	Ma		PC
Apparently drunk	R	R	Ma		Mi
Assault	R	R	Ma	Mi	Mi
Asthma	R	R	Ma		PC
Back pain	R	Ma		PC	PC
Behaving strangely	R			PA	■
Bites and stings	R	R	Ma		PC
Burns and scalds	R	R	Ma	Mi	Mi
Chest pain	R	R	Ma		PC
Collapsed adult	R	R	Ma		PC
Crying baby	R	R	Ma		PC
Dental problems	DC	DC	DC	DC	PC
Diabetes	R	R	Ma		PC
Diarrhoea and vomiting	R	R	Ma	PC	PC
Ear problems	R	R	Ma	PC	PC
Exposure to chemicals	R	R	Ma		PC
Eye problems	EC	EC	EC	EC	PC
Facial problems	R	R	Ma	Mi	Mi
Falls	R	R	Ma	Mi	Mi
Fits	R	R	Ma		PC
Foreign body	R	R	Ma		PC
GI bleeding	R	R	Ma		PC
Head injury	R	R	Ma	PC	PC
Headache	R	R	Ma	Mi	Mi
Irritable child	R	R	Ma	PC	PC
Limb problems	R	R		Mi	Mi
Limping child	R	R	Ma		PC
Major trauma	R	R	Ma	■	■
Mental illness	R			PA	■
Neck pain	R	R	Ma	Mi	Mi
Overdose and poisoning	R	R	Ma	PA	■
Palpitations	R	R	Ma		PC
Pregnancy	R	R	Ma		PC
PV bleeding	R	R	Ma		PC
Rashes	R	R	Ma		PC
Self-harm	R	R	Ma	Mi	■
Sexually acquired infection	R	R	SHC	SHC	SHC
Shortness of breath in adults	R	R	Ma		PC
Shortness of breath in children	R	R	Ma		PC
Sore throat	R	Ma	Ma	PC	PC
Testicular pain	R	Ma	Ma		PC
Torso injury	R	R	Ma	Mi	Mi

Continued

	1	2	3	4	5
Unwell adult	R	R	Ma	PC	PC
Unwell child	R	R	Ma		PC
Urinary problems	R	Ma	Ma		PC
Worried parent	R	R	Ma	PC	PC
Wounds	R	Ma		Mi	Mi

Key
DC   Emergency Dental provision
EC   Emergency Eye provision
Ma   Emergency Department Major Assessment
Mi   Minor Injuries provision
PA   Psychiatric Assessment
PC   Primary Care Emergency Centre
R   Emergency Department Resuscitation Area
SHC Sexual Health provision

Future uses

The Manchester Triage System has undoubtedly been used to assist in other processes within hospital and pre-hospital practice. Whenever any uses beyond prioritisation are considered it should always be remembered that the system was designed to prioritise Emergency Department patients. Any utility in processes other than this must be proved rather than assumed.

Presentational flow chart index

Continued

Presentational flow charts

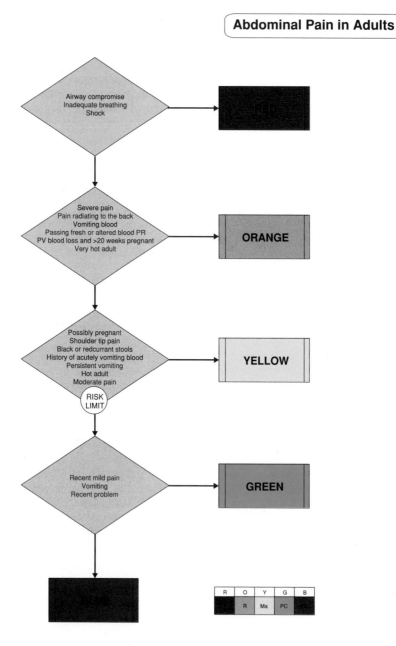

Abdominal Pain in Adults

Airway compromise Inadequate breathing Shock	→	RED		
Severe pain Pain radiating to the back Vomiting blood Passing fresh or altered blood PR PV blood loss and >20 weeks pregnant Very hot adult	→	**ORANGE**		
Possibly pregnant Shoulder tip pain Black or redcurrant stools History of acutely vomiting blood Persistent vomiting Hot adult Moderate pain RISK LIMIT	→	**YELLOW**		
Recent mild pain Vomiting Recent problem	→	**GREEN**		
BLUE				

R	O	Y	G	B
	R	Ma	PC	

Notes Accompanying Abdominal Pain in Adults

See also	Chart notes
GI bleeding, diarrhoea and vomiting, pregnancy	This is a presentation defined flow diagram. Abdominal pain is a common cause of presentation of surgical emergencies. A number of general discriminators are used including *Life Threat and Pain*. Specific discriminators are included in the ORANGE and YELLOW categories to ensure that the more severe pathologies are appropriately triaged. In particular discriminators are included to ensure that patients with moderate and severe GI bleeding and those with signs of retroperitoneal or diaphragmatic irritation are given sufficiently high categorisation

Specific discriminators	Explanation
Pain radiating to the back	Pain that is also felt in the back either intermittently of constantly
Vomiting blood	Vomited blood may be fresh (bright or dark red) or coffee ground in appearance
Passing fresh or altered blood PR	In active massive GI bleeding dark red blood will be passed PR. As GI transit time increases this becomes darker, eventually becoming melaena
PV blood loss and >20 weeks pregnant	Any loss of blood per vaginum in a woman known to be beyond the 20th week of pregnancy
Possibly pregnant	Any woman whose normal menstruation has failed to occur is possibly pregnant. Furthermore any woman of childbearing age who is having unprotected sex should be considered to be potentially pregnant
Shoulder tip pain	Pain felt in the tip of the shoulder. This often indicates diaphragmatic irritation
Black stool	Any blackness fulfils this criterion
Redcurrant stool	A dark red stool classically seen in intersussception
History of acutely vomiting blood	Frank haematemesis, vomiting of altered blood (coffee ground) or of blood mixed in the vomit within the past 24 hours
Persistent vomiting	Vomiting that is continuous or that occurs without any respite between episodes
Vomiting	Any emesis fulfils this criterion

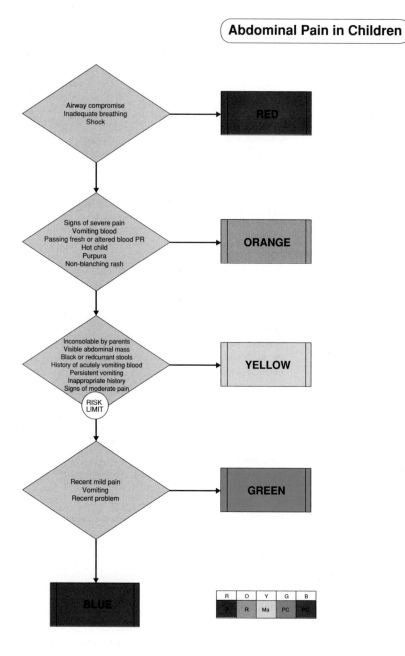

Abdominal Pain in Children

Airway compromise
Inadequate breathing
Shock

RED

Signs of severe pain
Vomiting blood
Passing fresh or altered blood PR
Hot child
Purpura
Non-blanching rash

ORANGE

Inconsolable by parents
Visible abdominal mass
Black or redcurrant stools
History of acutely vomiting blood
Persistent vomiting
Inappropriate history
Signs of moderate pain

RISK LIMIT

YELLOW

Recent mild pain
Vomiting
Recent problem

GREEN

BLUE

R	O	Y	G	B
R	R	Ma	PC	PC

Notes Accompanying Abdominal Pain in Children

See also	Chart notes
Diarrhoea and vomiting	This is a presentation defined flow diagram. Children who present with abdominal pain may have a range of pathologies and this chart has been designed to allow them to be accurately prioritised. A number of general discriminators are used including *Life Threat and Pain*. Specific discriminators are included to ensure the children who are actively bleeding, and those who have the signs or symptoms of more severe pathologies such as intersussception are seen urgently

Specific discriminators	Explanation
Signs of severe pain	Young children and babies in severe pain cannot complain. They will usually cry out continuously and inconsolably and be tachycardic. They may well exhibit signs such as pallor and sweating
Vomiting blood	Vomited blood may be fresh (bright or dark red) or coffee ground in appearance
Passing fresh or altered blood PR	In active massive GI bleeding dark red blood will be passed PR. As GI transit time increases this becomes darker, eventually becoming melaena
Purpura	A rash on any part of the body that is caused by small haemorrhages under the skin. A purpuric rash does not blanch (go white) when pressure is applied to it
Non-blanching rash	A rash that does not blanch (go white) when pressure is applied to it. Often tested using a glass tumbler to apply pressure as any colour change can be observed through the bottom of the tumbler
Signs of moderate pain	Young children and babies in moderate pain cannot complain. They will usually cry intermittently and are often intermittently consolable
Inconsolable by parents	Children whose crying or distress does not respond to attempts by their parents to comfort them fulfil this criterion
Visible abdominal mass	A mass in the abdomen that is visible to the naked eye
Black stool	Any blackness fulfils this criterion
Redcurrant stool	A dark red stool classically seen in intersussception. Absence of this type of stool does not rule out the diagnosis
Persistent vomiting	Vomiting that is continuous or that occurs without any respite
Inappropriate history	Children whose crying or distress does not respond to attempts by their parents to comfort them fulfil this criterion
Vomiting	Any emesis fulfils this criterion

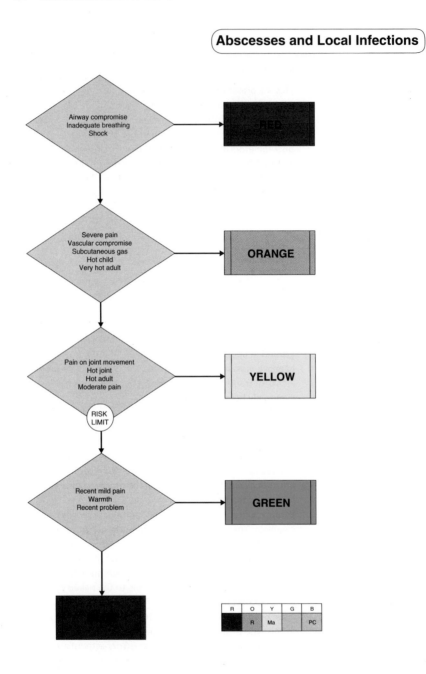

Notes Accompanying Abscessses and Local Infections

See also	Chart notes
Bites and stings	This is a presentation defined flow diagram designed to allow prioritisation of patients who present with a variety of obvious local infections and abscesses. Underlying conditions may vary from life threatening orbital cellulitis to acneiform spots. A number of general discriminators are used including *Life Threat, Pain and Temperature*. Specific discriminators have been included to allow identification of more urgent conditions such as gas gangrene and septic arthritis

Specific discriminators	Explanation
Vascular compromise	There will be a combination of pallor, coldness, altered sensation and pain with or without absent pulses distal to the injury
Subcutaneous gas	Gas under the skin can be detected by feeling for a 'crackling' on touch. There may be gas bubbles and a line of demarcation
Pain on joint movement	This can be pain on either active (patient) movement or passive (examiner) movement
Hot joint	Any warmth around a joint fulfils this criterion. Often accompanied by redness

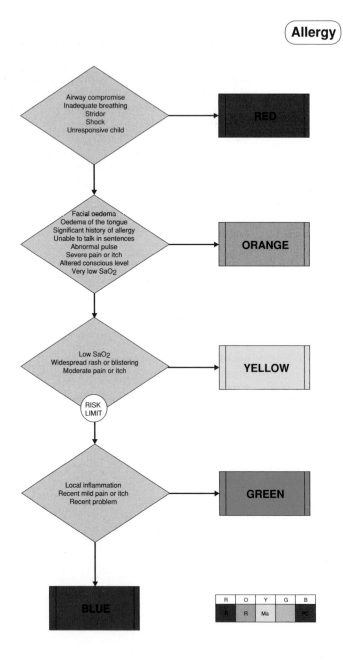

Allergy

RED
- Airway compromise
- Inadequate breathing
- Stridor
- Shock
- Unresponsive child

ORANGE
- Facial oedema
- Oedema of the tongue
- Significant history of allergy
- Unable to talk in sentences
- Abnormal pulse
- Severe pain or itch
- Altered conscious level
- Very low SaO$_2$

YELLOW
- Low SaO$_2$
- Widespread rash or blistering
- Moderate pain or itch

RISK LIMIT

GREEN
- Local inflammation
- Recent mild pain or itch
- Recent problem

BLUE

R	O	Y	G	B
R	R	Ma		PC

Notes Accompanying Allergy

See also	Chart notes
Collapsed adult, unwell adult, asthma, bites and stings	This is a presentation defined flow diagram designed to allow prioritisation of patients who present with symptoms and signs that may indicate allergy. The chart is a new chart, introduced in this edition at the request of users. Patients with allergic reactions range from those with life-threatening anaphylaxis to those with an itchy insect bite. A number of general discriminators are used including *Life Threat, Conscious Level and Pain*. Specific discriminators have been included to allow prioritisation of the most urgent conditions

Specific discriminators	Explanation
Facial oedema	Diffuse swelling around the face usually involving the lips
Oedema of the tongue	Swelling of the tongue of any degree
Significant history of allergy	A known sensitivity with severe reaction (e.g. to nuts or bee sting) is significant
Unable to talk in sentences	Patients who are so breathless that they cannot complete relatively short sentences in one breath
Abnormal pulse	A bradycardia (<60 min in adults), a tachycardia (>100 min in adults) or an irregular rhythm. Age appropriate definitions of bradycardia and tachycardia should be used in children
Very low SaO$_2$	This is a saturation <95% on O$_2$ therapy or <90% on air
Low SaO$_2$	This is a saturation of <95% on air
Widespread rash or blistering	Any discharging or blistering eruption covering more than 10% body surface area
Local inflammation	Local inflammation will involve pain, swelling and redness confined to a particular site or area

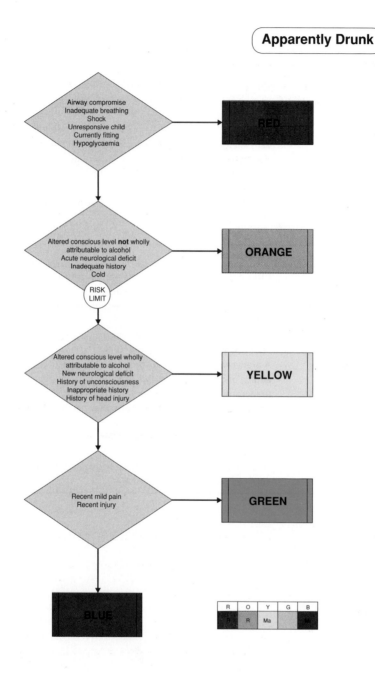

Apparently Drunk

Airway compromise
Inadequate breathing
Shock
Unresponsive child
Currently fitting
Hypoglycaemia

RED

Altered conscious level **not** wholly
attributable to alcohol
Acute neurological deficit
Inadequate history
Cold

RISK
LIMIT

ORANGE

Altered conscious level wholly
attributable to alcohol
New neurological deficit
History of unconsciousness
Inappropriate history
History of head injury

YELLOW

Recent mild pain
Recent injury

GREEN

BLUE

R	O	Y	G	B
P	R	Ma		

Notes Accompanying Apparently Drunk

See also	Chart notes
Behaving strangely Head injury Collapsed adult	This is a presentation defined flow diagram. A large number of patients attend for emergency treatment in an apparently drunken state. This chart implicitly recognises that not all these patients are drunk and is designed to ensure accurate identification and prioritisation of patients who are suffering from conditions which make them appear drunk, or from such severe drunkenness that their life is threatened. A number of general discriminators have been used including *Life Threat, Conscious Level in Children* and *Blood Glucose Level* A minor modification has been made to *Conscious Level in Adult* discriminator to ensure that only those adults who are unresponsive are placed into the very urgent category. However a specific discriminator is included to ensure that patients having an inadequate history of alcohol ingestion are seen rapidly and treated. If there is any doubt then the patient should be seen very urgently

Specific discriminators	Explanation
Altered conscious level *not* wholly attributable to alcohol	A patient who is not fully alert, with a history of alcohol ingestion, in whom there is any doubt at all that other causes of reduced conscious level may be present fulfils this discriminator definition
Acute neurological deficit	Any loss of neurological function that has come on within the previous 24 hours. This might include altered or lost sensation, weakness of the limbs (either transiently or permanently) and alterations in bladder or bowel function
Inadequate history	If there is no clear and unequivocal history of acute alcohol ingestion, and if head injury, drug ingestion, underlying medical condition, etc. cannot be definitely excluded then the history is inadequate
Altered conscious level wholly attributable to alcohol	A patient who is not fully alert, with a clear history of alcohol ingestion, and in whom there is no doubt that all other causes of reduced conscious level have been excluded fulfils this discriminator definition
New neurological deficit	Any loss of neurological function including altered or lost sensation, weakness of the limbs (either transiently or permanently) and alterations in bladder or bowel function
History of unconsciousness	There may be a reliable witness who can state whether the patient was unconscious (and for how long). If not a patient who is unable to remember the incident should be assumed to have been unconscious
Inappropriate history	When the history (story) given does not explain the physical findings it is termed inappropriate. This is important as it is a marker of non-accidental injury in vulnerable children and adults and may be the sentinel for abuse
History of head injury	A history of a recent physically traumatic event involving the head. Usually this will be reported by the patient but, if the patient has been unconscious this history should be sought from a reliable witness

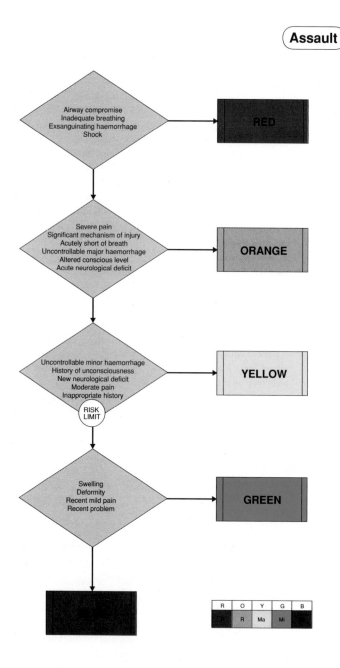

Notes Accompanying Assault

See also	Chart notes
Head injury, torso injury, wounds	This is a presentation defined flow diagram. Assault is a common presentation, and patients with non-specific conditions following assault may be triaged using this chart. Patients who have specific injuries are better triaged using the charts which pertain to those injuries. A number of general discriminators are used including *Life Threat, Haemorrhage and Pain*. Specific discriminators are included to identify patients who have a significant history of injury which may indicate a more urgent requirement for treatment

Specific discriminators	Explanation
Significant mechanism of injury	Penetrating injuries (stab or gunshot) and injuries with high energy transfer such as falls from heights and high speed road traffic accidents (speed > 40 mph) are significant especially if there has been ejection from the vehicle, the death(s) of other victim(s) of the accident or marked deformation of the vehicle
Acutely short of breath	Shortness of breath that comes on suddenly, or a sudden exacerbation of chronic shortness of breath
Acute neurological deficit	Any loss of neurological function that has come on within the previous 24 hours. This might include altered or lost sensation, weakness of the limbs (either transiently or permanently) and alterations in bladder or bowel function
History of unconsciousness	There may be a reliable witness who can state whether the patient was unconscious (and for how long). If not a patient who is unable to remember the incident should be assumed to have been unconscious
New neurological deficit	Any loss of neurological function including altered or lost sensation, weakness of the limbs (either transiently or permanently) and alterations in bladder or bowel function
Inappropriate history	When the history (story) given does not explain the physical findings it is termed inappropriate. This is important as it is a marker of non-accidental injury in vulnerable children and adults and may be the sentinel for abuse
Swelling	An abnormal increase in size
Deformity	This will always be subjective. Abnormal angulation or rotation is implied

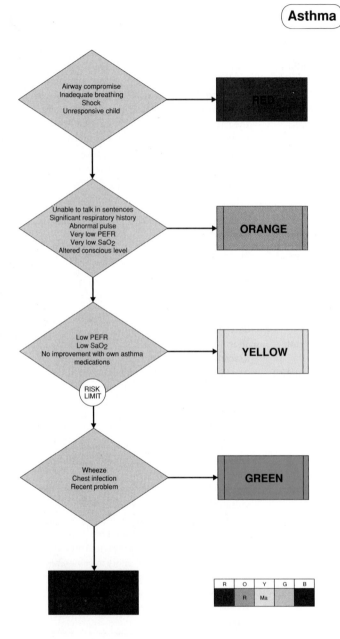

Asthma

Airway compromise
Inadequate breathing
Shock
Unresponsive child

RED

Unable to talk in sentences
Significant respiratory history
Abnormal pulse
Very low PEFR
Very low SaO$_2$
Altered conscious level

ORANGE

Low PEFR
Low SaO$_2$
No improvement with own asthma
medications

YELLOW

RISK
LIMIT

Wheeze
Chest infection
Recent problem

GREEN

R	O	Y	G	B
	R	Ma		

Notes Accompanying Asthma

See also	Chart notes
Shortness of breath in adults, shortness of breath in children, allergy	This is a presentation defined flow diagram which is intended for use in patients who present with the symptoms and signs of known asthma. The severity of asthmatic patients at presentation varies from those whose lives are threatened to those requiring a repeat prescription of inhalers. A number of general discriminators are used including *Life Threat, Conscious Level (in adults and children) and Oxygen Saturation*. Specific discriminators are included to indicate those signs and symptoms which indicate severe and life threatening asthma

Specific discriminators	Explanation
Unable to talk in sentences	Patients who are so breathless that they cannot complete relatively short sentences in one breath
Significant respiratory history	A history of previous life threatening episodes of a respiratory condition (eg COPD) is significant as is brittle asthma
Abnormal pulse	A bradycardia (<60 min in adults), a tachycardia (>100 min in adults) or an irregular rhythm. Age appropriate definitions of bradycardia and tachycardia should be used in children
Very low PEFR	This is a PEFR of 33% or less of best or predicted PEFR
Very low SaO_2	This is a saturation <95% on O_2 therapy or <90% on air
Low PEFR	This is a PEFR of 50% or less of best or predicted PEFR
Low SaO_2	This is a saturation of <95% on air
No improvement with own asthma medications	This history should be available from the patient. A failure to improve with bronchodilator therapy given by the GP or paramedic is equally significant
Wheeze	This can be audible wheeze or a feeling of wheeze. Very severe airway obstruction is silent (no air can move)
Chest infection	A chest infection usually causes a cough and production of sputum. This is usually purulent (green or yellow)

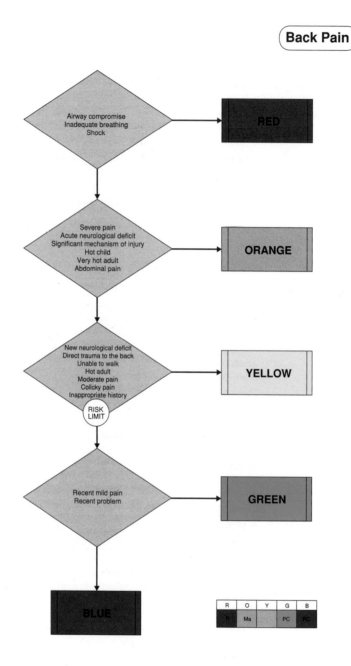

Back Pain

Notes Accompanying Back Pain

See also	Chart notes
Neck pain Abdominal pain	This is a presentation defined flow diagram. Back pain may present to the Emergency Department either as an acute event or as an acute exacerbation of the chronic problem. A number of general discriminators are used including *life threat, pain and temperature*. Specific discriminators have been selected in order to allow for appropriate categorisation of more urgent problems. In particular discriminators are included to allow appropriate classification of abdominal aneurysm, and patients with neurological signs and symptoms following disc prolapse

Specific discriminators	Explanation
Acute neurological deficit	Any loss of neurological function that has come on within the previous 24 hours. This might include altered or lost sensation, weakness of the limbs (either transiently or permanently) and alterations in bladder or bowel function
Significant mechanism of injury	Penetrating injuries (stab or gunshot) and injuries with high energy transfer such as falls from heights and high speed road traffic accidents (speed > 40 mph) are significant especially if there has been ejection from the vehicle; the death(s) of other victim(s) of the accident or marked deformation of the vehicle
Abdominal pain	Any pain felt in the abdomen. Abdominal pain associated with back pain may indicate abdominal aortic aneurysm, whilst association with PV bleeding may indicate ectopic pregnancy or miscarriage
New neurological deficit	Any loss of neurological function including altered or lost sensation, weakness of the limbs (either transiently or permanently) and alterations in bladder or bowel function
Direct trauma to the back	This may be top to bottom (loading) for instance when someone falls and lands on their feet, bending (forwards, backwards or to the side) or twisting
Unable to walk	It is important to try and distinguish between patients who have pain and difficulty walking, and those who *cannot* walk. Only the latter can be said to be unable to walk
Colicky pain	Pain that comes and goes in waves. Renal colic tends to come and go over 20 minutes or so
Inappropriate history	When the history (story) given does not explain the physical findings it is termed inappropriate. This is important as it is a marker of non-accidental injury in vulnerable children and adults and may be the sentinel for abuse

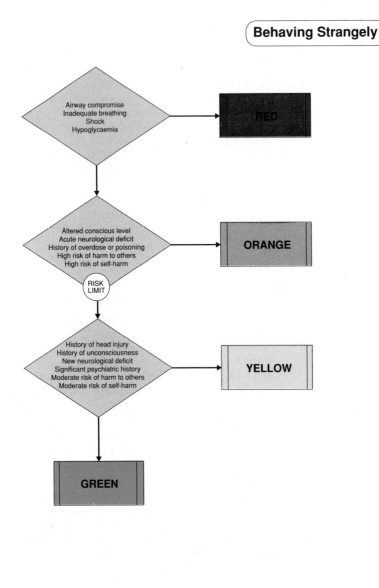

Behaving Strangely

Airway compromise
Inadequate breathing
Shock
Hypoglycaemia

RED

Altered conscious level
Acute neurological deficit
History of overdose or poisoning
High risk of harm to others
High risk of self-harm

ORANGE

RISK
LIMIT

History of head injury
History of unconsciousness
New neurological deficit
Significant psychiatric history
Moderate risk of harm to others
Moderate risk of self-harm

YELLOW

GREEN

R	O	Y	G	B
	Ma	Ma		

Notes Accompanying Behaving Strangely

See also	Chart notes
Apparently drunk Mental illness	This is a presentation defined flow diagram. Patients who are behaving strangely may have either a psychiatric or a physical cause for their presentation. This chart is designed to allow the accurate prioritisation of both these groups of patients. A number of general discriminators have been used including *Life Threat and Conscious Level*. Specific discriminators are used and in particular the concepts of risk of harm to others and risks of self-harm are introduced

Specific discriminators	Explanation
Hypoglycaemia	Glucose less than 3 mmol/l
Acute neurological deficit	Any loss of neurological function including altered or lost sensation, weakness of the limbs (either transiently or permanently) and alterations in bladder or bowel function
History of overdose or poisoning	This information may come from others or may be deduced if medication is missing
High risk of harm to others	The presence of a potential risk of harm to others can be judged by looking at posture (tense and clenched), speech patterns (loud and using threatening words) and motor behaviour (restless, pacing). High risk should be assumed if weapons and potential victims are available, or if self control is lost
High risk of self-harm	An initial view of the risk of self harm can be formed by considering the patients behaviour. Patients who have a significant history of self harm, are actively trying to harm themselves or who are actively trying to leave with the intent of harming themselves are at high risk
History of head injury	A history of a recent physically traumatic event involving the head. Usually this will be reported by the patient but if the patient has been unconscious this history should be sought from a reliable witness
History of unconsciousness	There may be a reliable witness who can state whether the patient was unconscious (and for how long). If not a patient who is unable to remember the incident should be assumed to have been unconscious
New neurological deficit	Any loss of neurological function including altered or lost sensation, weakness of the limbs (either transiently or permanently) and alterations in bladder or bowel function
Significant psychiatric history	A history of a major psychiatric illness or event
Moderate risk of harm to others	The presence of a potential risk of harm to others can be judged by looking at posture (tense and clenched), speech patterns (loud and using threatening words) and motor behaviour (restless, pacing). Moderate risk should be assumed if there is any indication of potential harm to others
Moderate risk of self-harm	An initial view of the risk of self-harm can be formed by considering the patients' behaviour. Patients without a significant history of self-harm, who are not actively trying to harm themselves, who are not actively trying to leave with the intent of harming themselves, but who profess the desire to harm themselves are at moderate risk

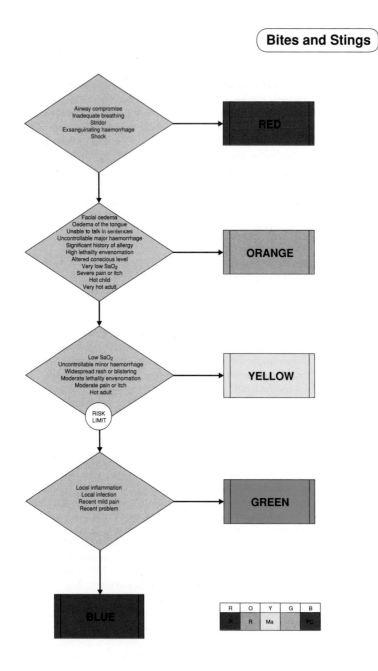

Bites and Stings

RED

Airway compromise
Inadequate breathing
Stridor
Exsanguinating haemorrhage
Shock

ORANGE

Facial oedema
Oedema of the tongue
Unable to talk in sentences
Uncontrollable major haemorrhage
Significant history of allergy
High lethality envenomation
Altered conscious level
Very low SaO_2
Severe pain or itch
Hot child
Very hot adult

YELLOW

Low SaO_2
Uncontrollable minor haemorrhage
Widespread rash or blistering
Moderate lethality envenomation
Moderate pain or itch
Hot adult

RISK LIMIT

GREEN

Local inflammation
Local infection
Recent mild pain
Recent problem

BLUE

R	O	Y	G	B
R	R	Ma		PC

Notes Accompanying Bites and Stings

See also	Chart notes
Allergy, abscesses and local infections	This is a presentation defined flow diagram designed to allow accurate prioritisation of patients who present following bites and stings. Bites may, of course, range from those delivered by insects to those delivered by large animals; therefore, there is a complete range of priority covered by this presentation. A number of general discriminators are used including *Life Threat, Haemorrhage and Pain*. Specific discriminators have been added to the chart to allow accurate identification of patients requiring more urgent treatment because of more severe injury or the development of allergic reactions

Specific discriminators	Explanation
Facial oedema	Diffuse swelling around the face usually involving the lips
Oedema of the tongue	Swelling of the tongue of any degree
Unable to talk in sentences	Patients who are so breathless that they cannot complete relatively short sentences in one breath
Significant history of allergy	A known sensitivity with severe reaction (e.g. to nuts or bee sting) is significant
High lethality envenomation	Lethality is the potential of the envenomation to cause harm. Local knowledge may allow identification of the venomous creature, but advice may be required. If in doubt assume a high risk
Very low SaO$_2$	This is a saturation <95% on O$_2$ therapy or <90% on air
Low SaO$_2$	This is a saturation of <95% on air
Widespread rash or itch	Any discharging or blistering eruption covering more than 10% body surface area
Moderate lethality envenomation	Lethality is the potential of the envenomation to cause harm. Local knowledge may allow identification of the venomous creature, but advice may be required
Local inflammation	Local inflammation will involve pain, swelling and redness confined to a particular site or area
Local infection	Local infection usually manifests as inflammation (pain, swelling and redness) confined to a particular site or area, with or without a collection of pus

Burns and Scalds

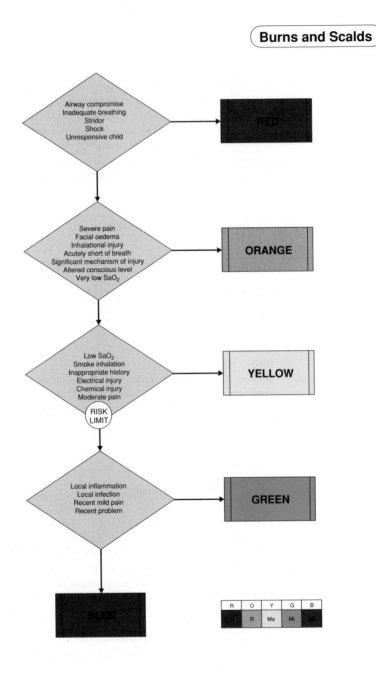

Notes Accompanying Burns and Scalds

See also	Chart notes
	This is a presentation defined flow diagram. There is a complete range of severity with this presentation and the chart has been designed to allow accurate identification of patients within each category. A number of general discriminators are used including *Life Threat, Conscious Level and Pain*. Specific discriminators have been added to allow identification of patients who have suffered inhalation injury, and those in whom the mechanism suggests that further investigation and treatment may be appropriate

Specific discriminators	Explanation
Facial oedema	Diffuse swelling around the face usually involving the lips
Inhalational injury	A history of being confined in a smoke filled space is the most reliable indicator of smoke inhalation. Carbon deposits around the mouth and nose and hoarse voice may be present. History is also the most reliable way of diagnosing inhalation of chemicals – there will not necessarily be any signs
Acutely short of breath	Shortness of breath that comes on suddenly, or a sudden exacerbation of chronic shortness of breath
Significant mechanism of injury	Penetrating injuries (stab or gunshot) and injuries with high energy transfer such as falls from heights and high speed road traffic accidents (speed $>$ 40 mph) are significant especially if there has been ejection from the vehicle, the death(s) of other victim(s) of the accident or marked deformation of the vehicle
Very low SaO_2	This is a saturation $<$95% on O_2 therapy or $<$90% on air
Low SaO_2	This is a saturation of $<$95% on air
Smoke inhalation	Smoke inhalation should be assumed if the patient has been confined in a smoke filled space. Physical signs such as oral or nasal soot are less reliable but significant if present
Inappropriate history	When the history (story) given does not explain the physical findings it is termed inappropriate. This is important as it is a marker of non-accidental injury in vulnerable children and adults and may be the sentinel for abuse
Electrical injury	Any injury caused or possibly caused by electric current. This includes AC and DC and both artificial and natural sources
Chemical injury	Any substance splashed onto or placed onto the body that causes stinging, burning, reduced vision or any other symptoms should be assumed to be capable of causing a chemical injury
Local inflammation	Local inflammation will involve pain, swelling and redness confined to a particular site or area
Local infection	Local infection usually manifests as inflammation (pain, swelling and redness) confined to a particular site or area, with or without a collection of pus

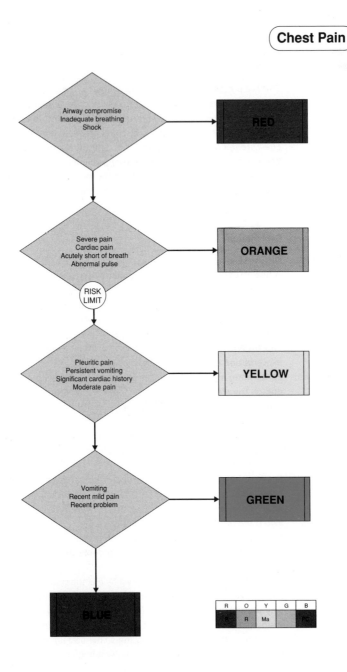

Chest Pain

RED

Airway compromise
Inadequate breathing
Shock

ORANGE

Severe pain
Cardiac pain
Acutely short of breath
Abnormal pulse

RISK
LIMIT

YELLOW

Pleuritic pain
Persistent vomiting
Significant cardiac history
Moderate pain

GREEN

Vomiting
Recent mild pain
Recent problem

BLUE

Notes Accompanying Chest Pain

See also	Chart notes
	This is a presentation defined flow diagram. Chest pain is a common presentation to Emergency Departments forming some 2–5% of all patient contacts. Causes of chest pain may vary from acute myocardial infraction to muscular irritation, and appropriate categorisation is paramount. A number of general discriminators are used including *Life Threat and Pain*. Specific discriminators include the nature and severity of pain (cardiac or pleuritic) and abnormalities of pulse

Specific discriminators	Explanation
Cardiac pain	Classically a severe dull 'gripping' or 'heavy' pain in the centre of the chest, radiating to the left arm or to the neck. May be associated with sweating and nausea
Acutely short of breath	Shortness of breath that comes on suddenly, or a sudden exacerbation of chronic shortness of breath
Abnormal pulse	A bradycardia (<60 min in adults), a tachycardia (>100 min in adults) or an irregular rhythm. Age appropriate definitions of bradycardia and tachycardia should be used in children
Pleuritic pain	A sharp, localised pain in the chest worse on breathing, coughing or sneezing
Persistent vomiting	Vomiting that is continuous or that occurs without any respite between episodes
Significant cardiac history	A known recurrent dysrhythmia which has life-threatening effects is significant as is a known cardiac condition that may deteriorate rapidly

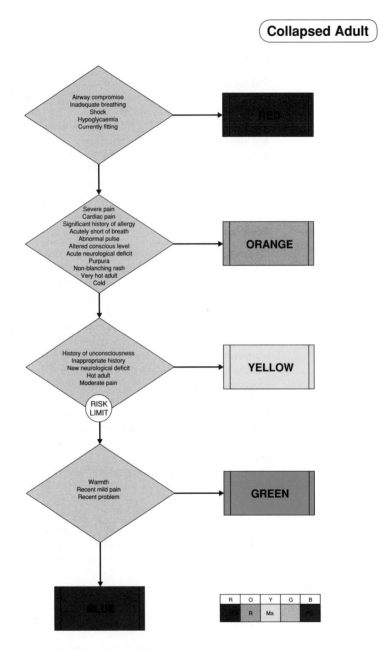

Collapsed Adult

Airway compromise
Inadequate breathing
Shock
Hypoglycaemia
Currently fitting

RED

Severe pain
Cardiac pain
Significant history of allergy
Acutely short of breath
Abnormal pulse
Altered conscious level
Acute neurological deficit
Purpura
Non-blanching rash
Very hot adult
Cold

ORANGE

History of unconsciousness
Inappropriate history
New neurological deficit
Hot adult
Moderate pain

YELLOW

RISK
LIMIT

Warmth
Recent mild pain
Recent problem

GREEN

BLUE

Notes Accompanying Collapsed Adult

See also	Chart notes
Fits Unwell Apparently drunk Falls	This is a presentation defined flow diagram. Presentation with collapse is not uncommon in an Emergency Department and this chart is designed to allow rapid triage of patients who present in this way. A number of general discriminators are used including *Life Threat, Conscious Level, Pain,* and *Temperature.* Specific discriminators have been added to the chart to try and rule out more serious pathology. As with all charts those pathologies (such as myocardial infarction) which can potentially benefit from early intervention are deliberately categorised highly

Specific discriminators	Explanation
Cardiac pain	Classically a severe dull 'gripping' or 'heavy' pain in the centre of the chest, radiating to the left arm or to the neck. May be associated with sweating and nausea
Significant history of allergy	A known sensitivity with severe reaction (e.g. to nuts or bee sting) is significant
Acutely short of breath	Shortness of breath that comes on suddenly, or a sudden exacerbation of chronic shortness of breath
Abnormal pulse	A bradycardia (<60 min in adults), a tachycardia (>100 min in adults) or an irregular rhythm. Age appropriate definitions of bradycardia and tachycardia should be used in children
Acute neurological deficit	Any loss of neurological function that has come on within the previous 24 hours. This might include altered or lost sensation, weakness of the limbs (either transiently or permanently) and alterations in bladder or bowel function
Purpura	A rash on any part of the body that is caused by small haemorrhages under the skin. A purpuric rash does not blanch (go white) when pressure is applied to it
Non-blanching rash	A rash that does not blanch (go white) when pressure is applied to it. Often tested using a glass tumbler to apply pressure as any colour change can be observed through the bottom of the tumbler
History of unconsciousness	There may be a reliable witness who can state whether the patient was unconscious (and for how long). If not a patient who is unable to remember the incident should be assumed to have been unconscious
Inappropriate history	When the history (story) given does not explain the physical findings it is termed inappropriate. This is important as it is a marker of non-accidental injury in vulnerable children and adults and may be the sentinel for abuse

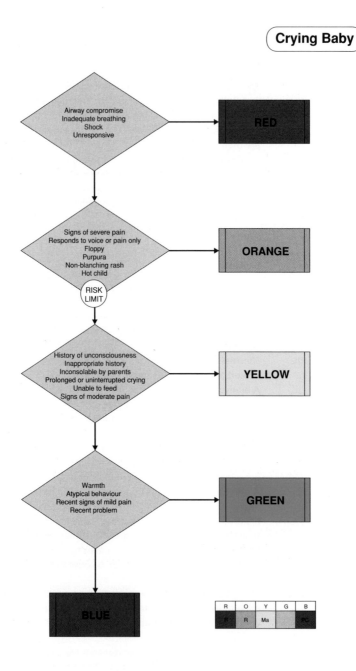

Crying Baby

Airway compromise
Inadequate breathing
Shock
Unresponsive

RED

Signs of severe pain
Responds to voice or pain only
Floppy
Purpura
Non-blanching rash
Hot child

ORANGE

RISK LIMIT

History of unconsciousness
Inappropriate history
Inconsolable by parents
Prolonged or uninterrupted crying
Unable to feed
Signs of moderate pain

YELLOW

Warmth
Atypical behaviour
Recent signs of mild pain
Recent problem

GREEN

BLUE

R	O	Y	G	B
R	R	Ma		PC

Notes Accompanying Crying Baby

See also	Chart notes
Unwell child, worried parent	This is a presentation defined flow diagram. This chart has been designed to allow accurate prioritisation of children who are presented by their parents with a chief complaint of crying. A number of general discriminators have been used including *Life Threat, Conscious Level and Pain*. Specific discriminators include those which allow recognition of more specific pathologies such as septicaemia, or which indicate that a more serious pathology might exist
	The risk limit sits between ORANGE and YELLOW and therefore no children can be categorised as YELLOW, GREEN or BLUE until all the specific and general discriminator outlined under the RED and ORANGE categories have been specifically excluded. This may take longer than the time available for initial assessment

Specific discriminators	Explanation
Signs of severe pain	Young children and babies in severe pain cannot complain. They will usually cry out continuously and inconsolably and be tachycardic. They may well exhibit signs such as pallor and sweating
Floppy	Parents may describe their children as floppy. Tone is generally reduced – the most noticeable sign is often lolling of the head
Purpura	A rash on any part of the body that is caused by small haemorrhages under the skin. A purpuric rash does not blanch (go white) when pressure is applied to it
Non-blanching rash	A rash that does not blanch (go white) when pressure is applied to it. Often tested using a glass tumbler to apply pressure as any colour change can be observed through the bottom of the tumbler
History of unconsciousness	There may be a reliable witness who can state whether the patient was unconscious (and for how long). If not a patient who is unable to remember the incident should be assumed to have been unconscious
Inappropriate history	When the history (story) given does not explain the physical findings it is termed inappropriate. This is important as it is a marker of non-accidental injury in vulnerable children and adults and may be the sentinel for abuse
Inconsolable by parents	Children whose crying or distress does not respond to attempts by their parents to comfort them fulfil this criterion
Prolonged or uninterrupted crying	A child who has cried continuously for 2 hours or more fulfils this criterion
Unable to feed	This is usually reported by the parents. Children who will not take any solid or liquid (as appropriate) by mouth
Signs of moderate pain	Young children and babies in moderate pain cannot complain. They will usually cry intermittently and are often intermittently consolable
Atypical behaviour	A child who is behaving in a way that is not usual in the given situation. The carers will often volunteer this information. Such children are often referred to as fractious or 'out of sorts'

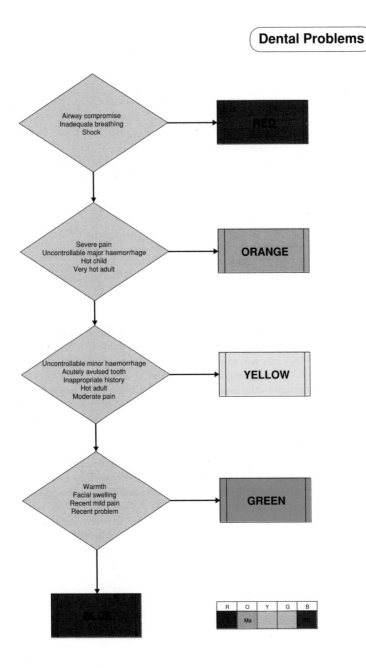

Dental Problems

Airway compromise
Inadequate breathing
Shock

RED

Severe pain
Uncontrollable major haemorrhage
Hot child
Very hot adult

ORANGE

Uncontrollable minor haemorrhage
Acutely avulsed tooth
Inappropriate history
Hot adult
Moderate pain

YELLOW

Warmth
Facial swelling
Recent mild pain
Recent problem

GREEN

BLUE

Notes Accompanying Dental Problems

See also	Chart notes
Facial problems	This is a presentation defined flow diagram designed to allow accurate prioritisation of patients presenting problems affecting the teeth or gums. A number of general discriminators have been used including *Life Threat, Pain, Haemorrhage and Temperature*. Acute avulsion of a tooth has been included in the very urgent (ORANGE) category since speed of reimplantation affects outcome It is important to ensure that preconceptions about disposal do not affect accurate triage of patients with these presentations

Specific discriminators	Explanation
Acutely avulsed tooth	A tooth that has been avulsed intact within the previous 24 hours
Inappropriate history	When the history (story) given does not explain the physical findings it is termed inappropriate. This is important as it is a marker of non-accidental injury in vulnerable children and adults and may be the sentinel for abuse
Facial swelling	Swelling around the face which may be localised or diffuse

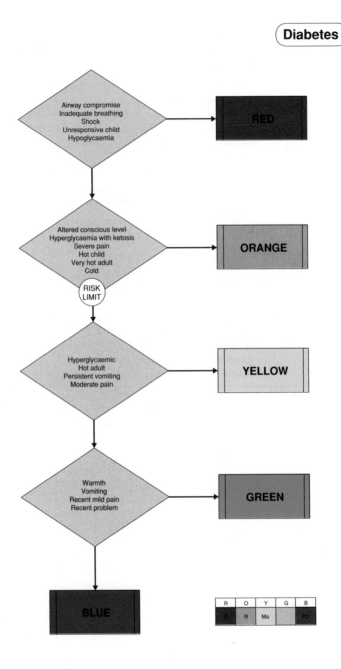

Diabetes

| Airway compromise
Inadequate breathing
Shock
Unresponsive child
Hypoglycaemia | RED |

| Altered conscious level
Hyperglycaemia with ketosis
Severe pain
Hot child
Very hot adult
Cold | ORANGE |

RISK LIMIT

| Hyperglycaemic
Hot adult
Persistent vomiting
Moderate pain | YELLOW |

| Warmth
Vomiting
Recent mild pain
Recent problem | GREEN |

BLUE

R	O	Y	G	B
R	R	Ma		PC

Notes Accompanying Diabetes

See also	Chart notes
	This is a presentation defined flow diagram designed to allow categorisation of patients who present with known cases of diabetes. A number of general discriminators are used including *Life Threat, Conscious Level (both adult and child), Blood Glucose Level and Temperature*

Specific discriminators	Explanation
Hypoglycaemia	Glucose less than 3 mmol/l
Hypoglycaemia with ketosis	Glucose greater than 11 mmol/l with urinary ketones or signs of acidosis (deep sighing respiration, etc.)
Hypoglycaemia	Glucose greater than 17 mmol/l
Persistent vomiting	Vomiting that is continuous or that occurs without any respite between episodes

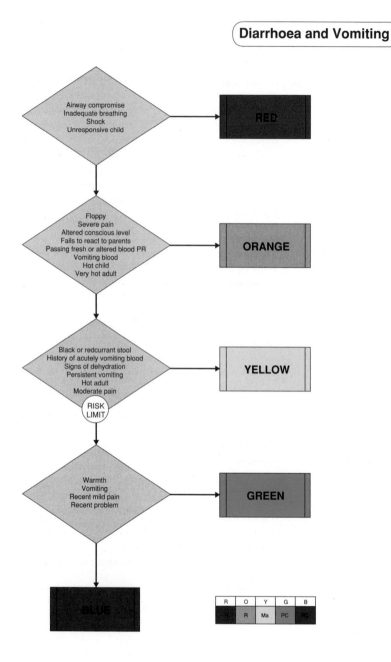

Diarrhoea and Vomiting

Airway compromise
Inadequate breathing
Shock
Unresponsive child

RED

Floppy
Severe pain
Altered conscious level
Fails to react to parents
Passing fresh or altered blood PR
Vomiting blood
Hot child
Very hot adult

ORANGE

Black or redcurrant stool
History of acutely vomiting blood
Signs of dehydration
Persistent vomiting
Hot adult
Moderate pain

YELLOW

RISK
LIMIT

Warmth
Vomiting
Recent mild pain
Recent problem

GREEN

BLUE

R	O	Y	G	B
RIS	R	Ma	PC	PC

Notes Accompanying Diarrhoea and Vomiting

See also	Chart notes
GI bleeding Abdominal pain in adults, abdominal pain in children	This is a new presentation defined flow diagram, combining the previous diarrhoea and vomiting charts. Most patients who present with diarrhoea or vomiting do not have high priority. However a number may have serious underlying pathology. A number of general discriminators are used including *Life Threat and Pain*. Specific discriminators have been included to ensure that patients suffering from GI bleeding, and those with dehydration and other severe effects of diarrhoea and vomiting are included in the appropriate categories

Specific discriminators	Explanation
Floppy	Parents may describe their children as floppy. Tone is generally reduced – the most noticeable sign is often lolling of the head
Fails to react to parents	Failure to react in any way to a parents' face or voice. Abnormal reactions and apparent lack of recognition of a parent are also worrying signs
Passing fresh or altered blood PR	In active massive GI bleeding dark red blood will be passed PR. As GI transit time increases this becomes darker, eventually becoming melaena
Vomiting blood	Vomited blood may be fresh (bright or dark red) or coffee ground in appearance
Black stool	Any blackness fulfils this criterion
Redcurrant stool	A dark red stool classically seen in intersussception
History of acutely vomiting blood	Frank haematemesis, vomiting of altered blood (coffee ground) or of blood mixed in the vomit within the past 24 hours
Signs of dehydration	These include dry tongue, sunken eyes, increased skin turgor and, in small babies, a sunken anterior fontanelle. Usually associated with a low urine output
Persistent vomiting	Vomiting that is continuous or that occurs without any respite between episodes

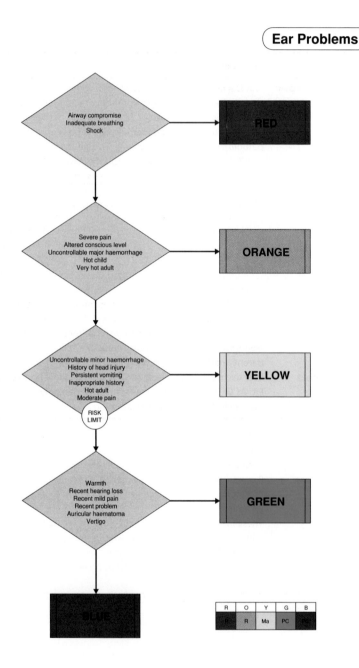

Ear Problems

Airway compromise
Inadequate breathing
Shock

RED

Severe pain
Altered conscious level
Uncontrollable major haemorrhage
Hot child
Very hot adult

ORANGE

Uncontrollable minor haemorrhage
History of head injury
Persistent vomiting
Inappropriate history
Hot adult
Moderate pain

RISK LIMIT

YELLOW

Warmth
Recent hearing loss
Recent mild pain
Recent problem
Auricular haematoma
Vertigo

GREEN

BLUE

R	O	Y	G	B
R	R	Ma	PC	PC

Notes Accompanying Ear Problems

See also	Chart notes
Facial problems, head injury	This is a presentation defined flow diagram designed to allow accurate prioritisation of patients presenting with conditions affecting the ear. A number of general discriminators are used including *Life Threat, Pain, Haemorrhage and Temperature*

Specific discriminators	Explanation
History of head injury	A history of a recent physically traumatic event involving the head. Usually this will be reported by the patient but if the patient has been unconscious this history should be sought from a reliable witness
Persistent vomiting	Vomiting that is continuous or that occurs without any respite between episodes
Inappropriate history	When the history (story) given does not explain the physical findings it is termed inappropriate. This is important as it is a marker of non-accidental injury in vulnerable children and adults and may be the sentinel for abuse
Recent hearing loss	Loss of hearing in one or both ears within the previous week
Auricular haematoma	A tense haematoma (usually post traumatic) in the outer ear
Vertigo	An acute feeling of spinning or dizziness, possibly accompanied by nausea and vomiting

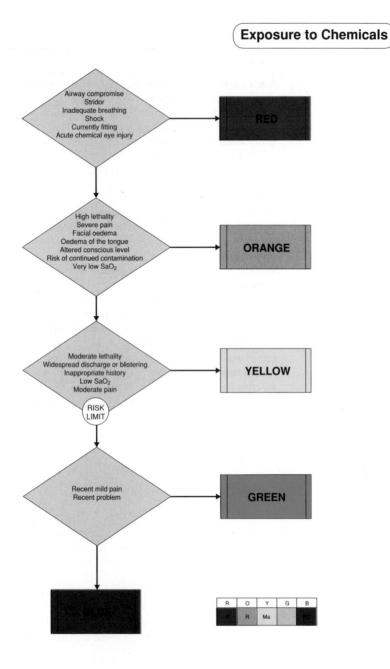

Exposure to Chemicals

Airway compromise
Stridor
Inadequate breathing
Shock
Currently fitting
Acute chemical eye injury

RED

High lethality
Severe pain
Facial oedema
Oedema of the tongue
Altered conscious level
Risk of continued contamination
Very low SaO$_2$

ORANGE

Moderate lethality
Widespread discharge or blistering
Inappropriate history
Low SaO$_2$
Moderate pain

YELLOW

RISK
LIMIT

Recent mild pain
Recent problem

GREEN

BLUE

R	O	Y	G	B
R	R	Ma		

Notes Accompanying Exposure to Chemicals

See also	Chart notes
Shortness of breath Shortness of breath in children Overdoses and poisoning	This is a presentation defined flow diagram. While this presentation is not common it is important because it is often the chief complaint of the patient. The signs and symptoms do not necessarily fit easily into any other presentational group. A number of general discriminators are used including *Life Threat, Conscious Level, Pain and Oxygen Saturation.* Specific discriminators which include those for the shortness of breath have been added to appropriate categories. *Acute Chemical Eye Injury* appears in the RED category and *Risk of Continued Contamination* appears in the ORANGE

Specific discriminators	Explanation
Stridor	This may be an inspiratory or expiratory noise, or both. Stridor is heard best on breathing with the mouth open
Acute chemical eye injury	Any substance splashed into or placed into the eye within the past 24 hours that caused stinging, burning or reduced vision should be assumed to be have caused chemical injury
High lethality	Lethality is the potential of the substance to which the casualty has been exposed to cause harm. Advice from a poisons centre may be required to establish the level of risk of serious illness or death. If in doubt assume a high risk
Facial oedema	Diffuse swelling around the face usually involving the lips
Oedema of the tongue	Swelling of the tongue of any degree
Risk of continued contamination	If chemical exposure is likely to continue (usually due to lack of adequate decontamination) then this discriminator applies. Risks to health care workers must not be forgotten if this situation occurs
Very low SaO_2	This is a saturation <95% on O_2 therapy or <90% on air
Moderate lethality	Lethality is the potential of the substance taken to cause serious illness or death. Advice from a poisons centre may be required to establish the level of risk to the patient
Widespread discharge or blistering	Any discharging or blistering eruption covering more than 10% body surface area
Inappropriate history	When the history (story) given does not explain the physical findings it is termed inappropriate. This is important as it is a marker of non-accidental injury in vulnerable children and adults and may be the sentinel for abuse
Low SaO_2	This is a saturation of <95% on air

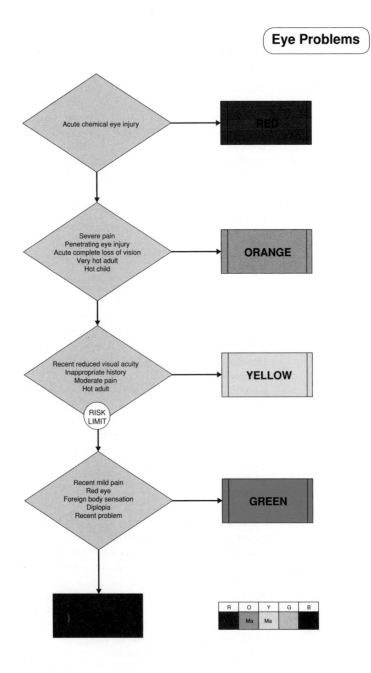

Eye Problems

Acute chemical eye injury → RED

Severe pain
Penetrating eye injury
Acute complete loss of vision
Very hot adult
Hot child
→ ORANGE

Recent reduced visual acuity
Inappropriate history
Moderate pain
Hot adult
→ YELLOW

RISK LIMIT

Recent mild pain
Red eye
Foreign body sensation
Diplopia
Recent problem
→ GREEN

R	O	Y	G	B
	Ma.	Ma		

Notes Accompanying Eye Problems

See also	Chart notes
Facial problems	This is a presentation defined flow diagram designed to allow accurate prioritisation of patients attending with conditions affecting the eye. *Pain* is used as a general discriminator. A number of specific discriminators have been used including a history of *acute chemical injury*, which indicates that immediate action is required, a history of *penetrating eye injury* or sudden or *acute complete loss of vision* and an assessment of visual acuity

Specific discriminators	Explanation
Acute chemical eye injury	Any substance splashed into or placed into the eye within the past 24 hours that caused stinging, burning or reduced vision should be assumed to have been caused chemical injury
Penetrating eye injury	A recent physically traumatic event involving penetration of the globe
Acute complete loss of vision	Loss of vision in one or both eyes within the preceding 24 hours which has not returned to normal
Recent reduced visual acuity	Any reduction in corrected visual acuity within the past 7 days
Inappropriate history	When the history (story) given does not explain the physical findings it is termed inappropriate. This is important as it is a marker of non-accidental injury in vulnerable children and adults and may be the sentinel for abuse
Red eye	Any redness to the eye. A red eye may be painful or painless and may be complete or partial
Foreign body sensation	A sensation of something in the eye, often expressed as scraping or grittiness
Diplopia	Double vision which resolves when one eye is closed

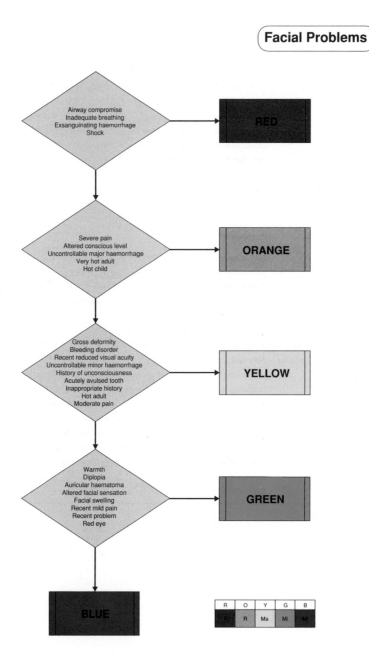

Facial Problems

Airway compromise		
Inadequate breathing		
Exsanguinating haemorrhage		
Shock	→	**RED**

Severe pain		
Altered conscious level		
Uncontrollable major haemorrhage	→	**ORANGE**
Very hot adult		
Hot child		

Gross deformity		
Bleeding disorder		
Recent reduced visual acuity		
Uncontrollable minor haemorrhage		
History of unconsciousness	→	**YELLOW**
Acutely avulsed tooth		
Inappropriate history		
Hot adult		
Moderate pain		

Warmth		
Diplopia		
Auricular haematoma		
Altered facial sensation		
Facial swelling	→	**GREEN**
Recent mild pain		
Recent problem		
Red eye		

BLUE

R	O	Y	G	B
Ru	R	Ma	Mi	Ml

Notes Accompanying Facial Problems

See also	Chart notes
Dental problems, ear problems, eye problems, head injury	This is a new presentation defined flow diagram which supersed the nasal problem chart. It has been designed to allow accurate prioritisation of patients attending with problems affecting the face. A number of general discriminators have been used including *Life Threat, Haemorrhage and Pain*

Specific discriminators	Explanation
Gross deformity	This will always be subjective. Gross and abnormal angulation or rotation is implied
Bleeding disorder	Congenital or acquired bleeding disorder
Recent reduced visual acuity	Any reduction in corrected visual acuity within the past 7 days
History of unconsciousness	There may be a reliable witness who can state whether the patient was unconscious (and for how long). If not a patient who is unable to remember the incident should be assumed to have been unconscious
Acutely avulsed tooth	A tooth that has been avulsed intact within the previous 24 hours
Inappropriate history	When the history (story) given does not explain the physical findings it is termed inappropriate. This is important as it is a marker of non-accidental injury in vulnerable children and adults and may be the sentinel for abuse
Diplopia	Double vision which resolves when one eye is closed
Auricular haematoma	A tense haematoma (usually post traumatic) in the outer ear
Altered facial sensation	Any alteration of sensation on the face
Facial swelling	Swelling around the face which may be localised or diffuse
Red eye	Any redness to the eye. A red eye may be painful or painless and may be complete or partial

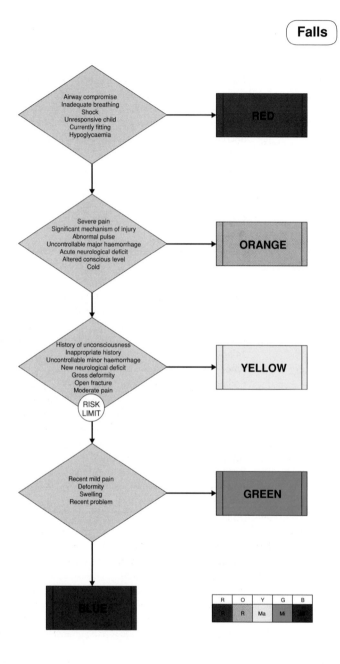

Notes Accompanying Falls

See also	Chart notes
Collapsed adult	This is a presentation defined flow diagram. Many patients who present with a history of falls have suffered trauma as a result, and their priority will reflect the injuries suffered. Some, however, may have had a serious underlying pathology which has caused them to fall, or may have developed complications after falling. This chart is designed to allow accurate prioritisation whether the injury or underlying cause is more pressing. A number of general discriminators have been included to ensure that patients suffering from serious underlying conditions or limb threatening injuries are given a high priority

Specific discriminators	Explanation
Hypoglycaemia	Glucose less than 3 mmol/l
Significant mechanism of injury	Penetrating injuries (stab or gunshot) and injuries with high energy transfer such as falls from heights and high speed road traffic accidents (speed > 40 mph) are significant especially if there has been ejection from the vehicle, the death(s) of other victim(s) of the accident or marked deformation of the vehicle
Abnormal pulse	A bradycardia (<60 min in adults), a tachycardia (>100 min in adults) or an irregular rhythm. Age appropriate definitions of bradycardia and tachycardia should be used in children
Acute neurological deficit	Any loss of neurological function that has come on within the previous 24 hours. This might include altered or lost sensation, weakness of the limbs (either transiently or permanently) and alterations in bladder or bowel function
History of unconsciousness	There may be a reliable witness who can state whether the patient was unconscious (and for how long). If not a patient who is unable to remember the incident should be assumed to have been unconscious
Inappropriate history	When the history (story) given does not explain the physical findings it is termed inappropriate. This is important as it is a marker of non-accidental injury in vulnerable children and adults and may be the sentinel for abuse
New neurological deficit	Any loss of neurological function including altered or lost sensation, weakness of the limbs (either transiently or permanently) and alterations in bladder or bowel function
Gross deformity	This will always be subjective. Gross and abnormal angulation or rotation is implied
Open fracture	All wounds in the vicinity of a fracture should be regarded with suspicion. If there is any possibility of communication between the wound and the fracture then the fracture should be assumed to be open
Deformity	This will always be subjective. Abnormal angulation or rotation is implied
Swelling	An abnormal increase in size

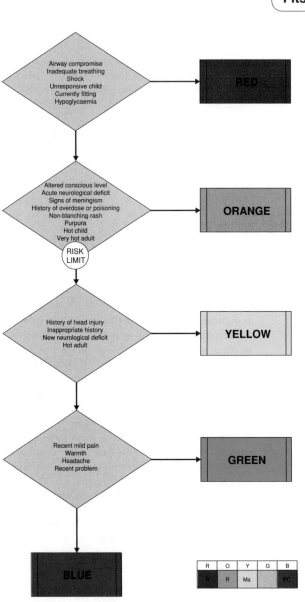

Fits

Airway compromise
Inadequate breathing
Shock
Unresponsive child
Currently fitting
Hypoglycaemia

RED

Altered conscious level
Acute neurological deficit
Signs of meningism
History of overdose or poisoning
Non-blanching rash
Purpura
Hot child
Very hot adult
RISK LIMIT

ORANGE

History of head injury
Inappropriate history
New neurological deficit
Hot adult

YELLOW

Recent mild pain
Warmth
Headache
Recent problem

GREEN

BLUE

R	O	Y	G	B
R	R	Ma		PC

Notes Accompanying Fits

See also	Chart notes
Head injury Headache Overdoses and poisoning	This is a presentation defined flow diagram. It is not an uncommon presentation to the Emergency Department and this chart is designed to allow rapid categorisation of patients who are currently fitting or who have fitted. A number of general discriminators are used including life threat, conscious level and temperature. Specific discriminators include signs of meningism and a focal or progressive loss of function As with all unconscious patients rapid blood sugar estimation would be indicated to exclude hypoglycaemia

Specific discriminators	Explanation
Currently fitting	Patients who are in the tonic or clonic stages of a grand mal convulsion, and patients currently experiencing partial fits fulfil this criterion
Hypoglycaemia	Glucose less than 3 mmol/l
Acute neurological deficit	Any loss of neurological function that has come on within the previous 24 hours. This might include altered or lost sensation, weakness of the limbs (either transiently or permanently) and alterations in bladder or bowel function
Signs of meningism	Classically a stiff neck together with headache and photophobia
History of overdose or poisoning	This information may come from others or may be deduced if medication is missing
Non-blanching rash	A rash that does not blanch (go white) when pressure is applied to it. Often tested using a glass tumbler to apply pressure as any colour change can be observed through the bottom of the tumbler
Purpura	A rash on any part of the body that is caused by small haemorrhages under the skin. A purpuric rash does not blanch (go white) when pressure is applied to it
History of head injury	A history of a recent physically traumatic event involving the head. Usually this will be reported by the patient but if the patient has been unconscious this history should be sought from a reliable witness
Inappropriate history	When the history (story) given does not explain the physical findings it is termed inappropriate. This is important as it is a marker of non-accidental injury in vulnerable children and adults and may be the sentinel for abuse
New neurological deficit	Any loss of neurological function including altered or lost sensation, weakness of the limbs (either transiently or permanently) and alterations in bladder or bowel function
Headache	Any pain around the head that is not related to a particular anatomical structure. Facial pain is not included

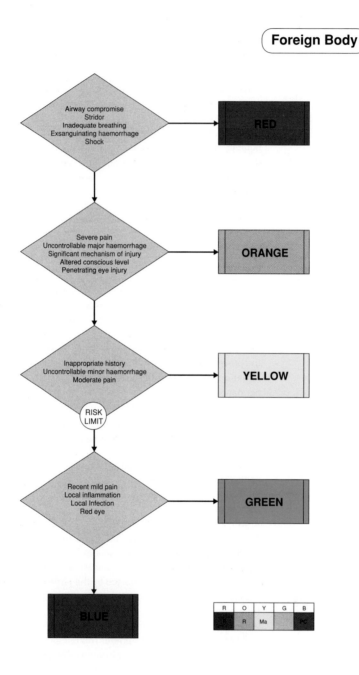

Notes Accompanying Foreign Body

See also	Chart notes
Wounds, torso injury	This is a presentation defined flow diagram designed to allow accurate prioritisation of patients who present with foreign bodies in any part of their anatomy. The severity of such cases can range from the inconvenient to the life threatening and this chart is designed to differentiate between these. A number of general discriminators have been used including *Life Threat, Haemorrhage and Pain*. The only specific discriminator that relates to anatomical site is that of eye penetration

Specific discriminators	Explanation
Stridor	This may be an inspiratory or expiratory noise, or both. Stridor is heard best on breathing with the mouth open
Significant mechanism of injury	Penetrating injuries (stab or gunshot) and injuries with high energy transfer such as falls from heights and high speed road traffic accidents (speed > 40 mph) are significant especially if there has been ejection from the vehicle, the death(s) of other victim(s) of the accident or marked deformation of the vehicle
Penetrating eye injury	A recent physically traumatic event involving penetration of the globe
Inappropriate history	When the history (story) given does not explain the physical findings it is termed inappropriate. This is important as it is a marker of non-accidental injury in vulnerable children and adults and may be the sentinel for abuse
Local inflammation	Local inflammation will involve pain, swelling and redness confined to a particular site or area
Local infection	Local infection usually manifests as inflammation (pain, swelling and redness) confined to a particular site or area, with or without a collection of pus
Red eye	Any redness to the eye. A red eye may be painful or painless and may be complete or partial

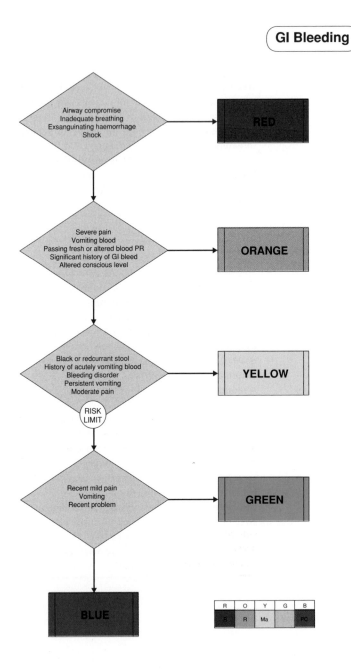

Notes Accompanying GI Bleeding

See also	Chart notes
Diarrhoea and vomiting, abdominal pain in adults, abdominal pain in children	This is a presentation defined flow diagram. Patients may present with GI bleeding either as vomiting altered or unaltered blood, or by passing blood PR. A number of general discriminators are used including *Life Threat* and *Pain*. Specific discriminators have been selected to indicate the current severity of the GI bleeding. Thus patients vomiting blood or those passing fresh or altered blood PR have a higher category than those with a history of vomiting

Specific discriminators	Explanation
Vomiting blood	Vomited blood may be fresh (bright or dark red) or coffee ground in appearance
Passing fresh or altered blood PR	In active massive GI bleeding dark red blood will be passed PR. As GI transit time increases this becomes darker, eventually becoming melaena
Significant history of GI bleed	Any history of massive GI bleeding or of any GI bleed associated with oesophageal varices
Black stool	Any blackness fulfils this criterion
Redcurrant stool	A dark red stool classically seen in intersussception
History of acutely vomiting blood	Frank haematemesis, vomiting of altered blood (coffee ground) or of blood mixed in the vomit within the past 24 hours
Bleeding disorder	Any blackness fulfils this criterion
Persistent vomiting	Vomiting that is continuous or that occurs without any respite between episodes

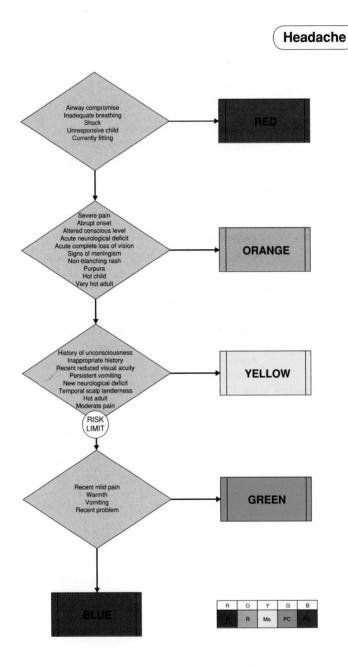

Notes Accompanying Headache

See also	Chart notes
Head injury Neck pain	This is a presentation defined flow diagram. A large number of conditions can present with headache and a number of these require urgent intervention. A number of general discriminators are used including *Life Threat, Conscious Level, Pain and Temperature*. Specific discriminators have been used to identify severe causes such as subarachnoid haemorrhage and meningococcocaemia. New neurological signs or symptoms together with reduction in visual acuity and tenderness of the scalp are used to indicate the need for urgent clinical review

Specific discriminators	Explanation
Currently fitting	Patients who are in the tonic or clonic stages of a grand mal convulsion, and patients currently experiencing partial fits fulfil this criterion
Abrupt onset	Onset within seconds or minutes. May cause waking from sleep
Acute neurological deficit	Any loss of neurological function that has come on within the previous 24 hours. This might include altered or lost sensation, weakness of the limbs (either transiently or permanently) and alterations in bladder or bowel function
Acute complete loss of vision	Loss of vision in one or both eyes within the preceding 24 hours which has not returned to normal
Signs of meningism	Classically a stiff neck together with headache and photophobia
Non-blanching rash	A rash that does not blanch (go white) when pressure is applied to it. Often tested using a glass tumbler to apply pressure as any colour change can be observed through the bottom of the tumbler
Purpura	A rash on any part of the body that is caused by small haemorrhages under the skin. A purpuric rash does not blanch (go white) when pressure is applied to it
History of unconsciousness	There may be a reliable witness who can state whether the patient was unconscious (and for how long). If not a patient who is unable to remember the incident should be assumed to have been unconscious
Inappropriate history	When the history (story) given does not explain the physical findings it is termed inappropriate. This is important as it is a marker of non-accidental injury in vulnerable children and adults and may be the sentinel for abuse
Recent reduced visual acuity	Any reduction in corrected visual acuity within the past 7 days
Persistent vomiting	Vomiting that is continuous or that occurs without any respite between episodes
New neurological deficit	Any loss of neurological function including altered or lost sensation, weakness of the limbs (either transiently or permanently) and alterations in bladder or bowel function
Temporal scalp tenderness	Tenderness on palpation over the temporal area (especially over the artery)

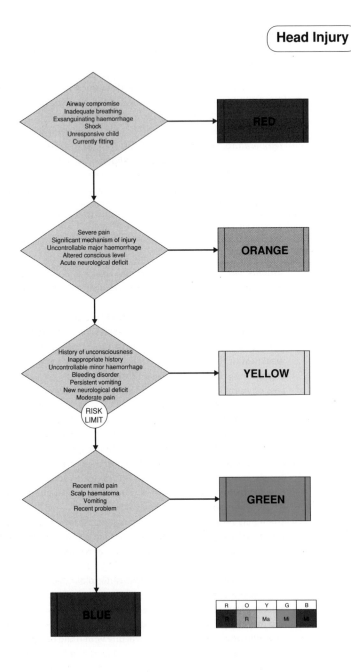

Head Injury

Airway compromise
Inadequate breathing
Exsanguinating haemorrhage
Shock
Unresponsive child
Currently fitting

RED

Severe pain
Significant mechanism of injury
Uncontrollable major haemorrhage
Altered conscious level
Acute neurological deficit

ORANGE

History of unconsciousness
Inappropriate history
Uncontrollable minor haemorrhage
Bleeding disorder
Persistent vomiting
New neurological deficit
Moderate pain

RISK LIMIT

YELLOW

Recent mild pain
Scalp haematoma
Vomiting
Recent problem

GREEN

BLUE

R	O	Y	G	B
R	R	Ma	Mi	Mi

Notes Accompanying Head Injury

See also	Chart notes
Headache, neck pain, fits	This is a presentation defined flow diagram. Head injury is an extremely common presentation and its effects may vary from life threatening extradural haemorrhage to minimal scalp injury. A number of general discriminators have been used including *Life Threat, Conscious Level (both in adults and children), Haemorrhage and Pain*. Specific discriminators are included to select those patients with significant mechanism and the development of neurological signs and symptoms, to a higher priority

Discriminators	Explanation
Currently fitting	Patients who are in the tonic or clonic stages of a grand mal convulsion, and patients currently experiencing partial fits fulfil this criterion
Significant mechanism of injury	Penetrating injuries (stab or gunshot) and injuries with high energy transfer such as falls from heights and high speed road traffic accidents (speed > 40 mph) are significant especially if there has been ejection from the vehicle, death(s) of other victim(s) of the accident or marked deformation of the vehicle
Acute neurological deficit	Any loss of neurological function that has come on within the previous 24 hours. This might include altered or lost sensation, weakness of the limbs (either transiently or permanently) and alterations in bladder or bowel function
History of unconsciousness	There may be a reliable witness who can state whether the patient was unconscious (and for how long). If not a patient who is unable to remember the incident should be assumed to have been unconscious
Inappropriate history	When the history (story) given does not explain the physical findings it is termed inappropriate. This is important as it is a marker of non-accidental injury in vulnerable children and adults and may be the sentinel for abuse
Bleeding disorder	Congenital or acquired bleeding disorder
Persistent vomiting	Vomiting that is continuous or that occurs without any respite between episodes
New neurological deficit	Any loss of neurological function including altered or lost sensation, weakness of the limbs (either transiently or permanently) and alterations in bladder or bowel function
Scalp haematoma	A raised bruised area to the scalp (bruises below the hair line at the front are to the forehead

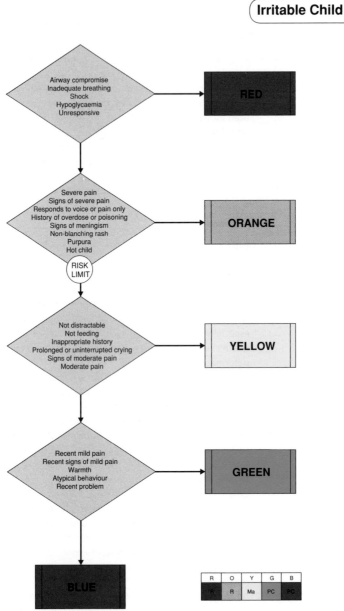

Irritable Child

Airway compromise
Inadequate breathing
Shock
Hypoglycaemia
Unresponsive

RED

Severe pain
Signs of severe pain
Responds to voice or pain only
History of overdose or poisoning
Signs of meningism
Non-blanching rash
Purpura
Hot child

RISK
LIMIT

ORANGE

Not distractable
Not feeding
Inappropriate history
Prolonged or uninterrupted crying
Signs of moderate pain
Moderate pain

YELLOW

Recent mild pain
Recent signs of mild pain
Warmth
Atypical behaviour
Recent problem

GREEN

BLUE

R	O	Y	G	B
R	R	Ma	PC	PC

Notes Accompanying Irritable Child

See also	Chart notes
Crying baby, unwell child, worried parent	This is a presentation defined flow diagram. It is designed to be used in children over the age of 1 year. A number of general discriminators have been used including *Life Threat, Conscious Level and Pain*. Specific discriminators include those which allow recognition of more specific pathologies such as septicaemia, or which indicate that a more serious pathology might exist
	The risk limit sits between ORANGE and YELLOW and therefore no children can be categorised as YELLOW, GREEN or BLUE until all the specific and general discriminators outlined under the RED and ORANGE categories have been specifically excluded. This may take longer than the time available for initial assessment

Specific discriminators	Explanation
Hypoglycaemia	Glucose less than 3 mmol/l
Signs of severe pain	Young children and babies in severe pain cannot complain. They will usually cry out continuously and inconsolably and be tachycardic. They may well exhibit signs such as pallor and sweating
History of overdose or poisoning	This information may come from others or may be deduced if medication is missing
Signs of meningism	Classically a stiff neck together with headache and photophobia
Non-blanching rash	A rash that does not blanch (go white) when pressure is applied to it. Often tested using a glass tumbler to apply pressure as any colour change can be observed through the bottom of the tumbler
Purpura	A rash on any part of the body that is caused by small haemorrhages under the skin. A purpuric rash does not blanch (go white) when pressure is applied to it
Not distractable	Children who are distressed by pain or other things who cannot be distracted by conversation or play fulfil this criterion
Not feeding	Children who will not take any solid or liquid (as appropriate) by mouth. Children who will take the food but always vomit afterwards may also fulfil this criterion
Inappropriate history	When the history (story) given does not explain the physical findings it is termed inappropriate. This is important as it is a marker of non-accidental injury in vulnerable children and adults and may be the sentinel for abuse
Prolonged or uninterrupted crying	A child who has cried continuously for 2 hours or more fulfils this criterion
Signs of moderate pain	Young children and babies in moderate pain cannot complain. They will usually cry intermittently and are often intermittently consolable
Atypical behaviour	A child who is behaving in a way that is not usual in the given situation. The carers will often volunteer this information. Such children are often referred to as fractious or 'out of sorts'

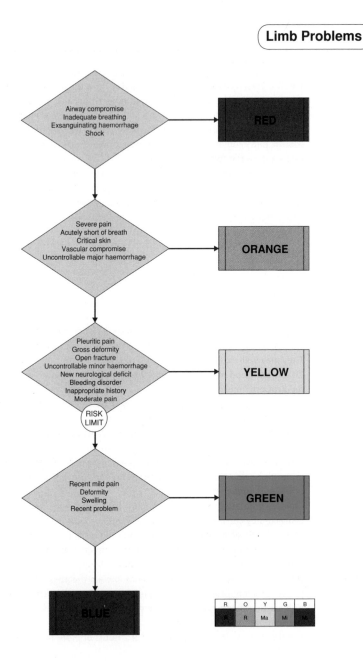

Limb Problems

| Airway compromise
Inadequate breathing
Exsanguinating haemorrhage
Shock | → | **RED** |

| Severe pain
Acutely short of breath
Critical skin
Vascular compromise
Uncontrollable major haemorrhage | → | **ORANGE** |

| Pleuritic pain
Gross deformity
Open fracture
Uncontrollable minor haemorrhage
New neurological deficit
Bleeding disorder
Inappropriate history
Moderate pain | → | **YELLOW** |

RISK LIMIT

| Recent mild pain
Deformity
Swelling
Recent problem | → | **GREEN** |

BLUE

R	O	Y	G	B
R	R	Ma	Mi	Mi

Notes Accompanying Limb Problems

See also	Chart notes
Limping child	This is a presentation defined flow diagram. Injuries to the limbs are the commonest presentation to Emergency Departments and, while rarely life threatening, may cause considerable morbidity. A number of general discriminators are used including *Life Threat, Haemorrhage and Pain*. Specific discriminators are included to ensure that limb threatening injuries are seen and treated urgently. Discriminators are also included to remind the triage practitioner to consider the signs and symptoms of thromboembolic disease and its complications

Specific discriminators	Explanation
Acutely short of breath	Shortness of breath that comes on suddenly, or a sudden exacerbation of chronic shortness of breath
Critical skin	A fracture or dislocation may leave fragments or ends of bone pressing so hard against the skin that the viability of the skin is threatened. The skin will be white and under tension
Vascular compromise	There will be a combination of pallor, coldness, altered sensation and pain with or without absent pulses distal to the injury
Pleuritic pain	A sharp, localised pain in the chest made worse on breathing, coughing or sneezing
Gross deformity	This will always be subjective. Gross and abnormal angulation or rotation is implied
Open fracture	All wounds in the vicinity of a fracture should be regarded with suspicion. if there is any possibility of communication between the wound and the fracture then the fracture should be assumed to be open
New neurological deficit	Any loss of neurological function including altered or lost sensation, weakness of the limbs (either transiently or permanently) and alterations in bladder or bowel function
Bleeding disorder	Congenital or acquired bleeding disorder
Inappropriate history	When the history (story) given does not explain the physical findings it is termed inappropriate. This is important as it is a marker of non-accidental injury in vulnerable children and adults and may be the sentinel for abuse
Deformity	This will always be subjective. Abnormal angulation or rotation is implied
Swelling	An abnormal increase in size

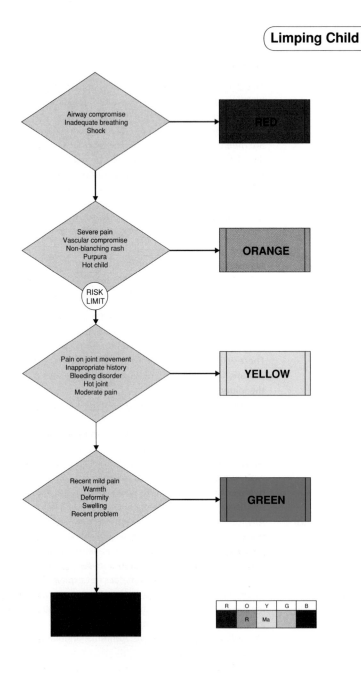

Limping Child

Airway compromise
Inadequate breathing
Shock

RED

Severe pain
Vascular compromise
Non-blanching rash
Purpura
Hot child

ORANGE

RISK
LIMIT

Pain on joint movement
Inappropriate history
Bleeding disorder
Hot joint
Moderate pain

YELLOW

Recent mild pain
Warmth
Deformity
Swelling
Recent problem

GREEN

R	O	Y	G	B
	R	Ma		

Notes Accompanying Limping Child

See also	Chart notes
Limb injuries	This is a presentation defined flow diagram. Children who present with limp range from those who have suffered a minor soft tissue injury to the foot or ankle to those who have developed septic arthritis of the hip. This chart is designed to allow accurate prioritisation of such children. A number of general discriminators are used including *Life Threat, Pain and Temperature*. Specific discriminators have been included to allow children with more urgent pathologies which threaten distal function from being accurately identified, and those in whom the limp is a sinister sign of systemic disease from being spotted quickly The risk limit sits between ORANGE and YELLOW and therefore no children can be categorised as YELLOW, GREEN or BLUE until all the specific and general discriminators outlined under the RED and ORANGE categories have been specifically excluded. This may take longer than the time available for initial assessment

Specific discriminators	Explanation
Vascular compromise	There will be a combination of pallor, coldness, altered sensation and pain with or without absent pulses distal to the injury
Non-blanching rash	A rash that does not blanch (go white) when pressure is applied to it. Often tested using a glass tumbler to apply pressure as any colour change can be observed through the bottom of the tumbler
Purpura	A rash on any part of the body that is caused by small haemorrhages under the skin. A purpuric rash does not blanch (go white) when pressure is applied to it
Pain on joint movement	This can be pain on either active (patient) movement or passive (examiner) movement
Inappropriate history	When the history (story) given does not explain the physical findings it is termed inappropriate
Bleeding disorder	This is important as it is a marker of non-accidental injury in vulnerable children and adults and may be the sentinel for abuse
Hot joint	Any warmth around a joint fulfils this criterion. Often accompanied by redness
Deformity	This will always be subjective. Abnormal angulation or rotation is implied
Swelling	An abnormal increase in size

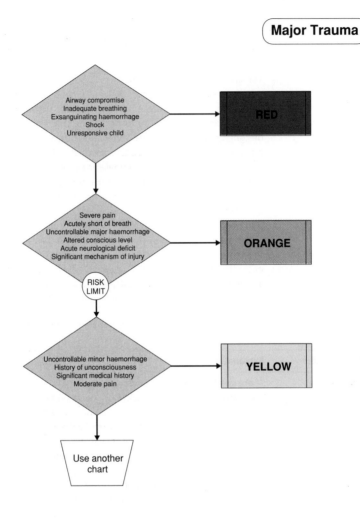

Major Trauma

Airway compromise
Inadequate breathing
Exsanguinating haemorrhage
Shock
Unresponsive child

RED

Severe pain
Acutely short of breath
Uncontrollable major haemorrhage
Altered conscious level
Acute neurological deficit
Significant mechanism of injury

ORANGE

RISK
LIMIT

Uncontrollable minor haemorrhage
History of unconsciousness
Significant medical history
Moderate pain

YELLOW

Use another
chart

Notes Accompanying Major Truma

See also	Chart notes
	Most health care providers know what is implied by major trauma but it is a strange presentation in that it is defined not by the patients or their injury, but on some judgement of that injury by the carers. For this reason it is impossible to categorise a patient with this presentation as less than urgent. If it is necessary to do this then a deliberate decision needs to be made that the original description of the patient as having suffered major trauma was incorrect, and the patient should be categorised using a different presentational flow diagram
	A number of general discriminators have been used including *Life Threat, Haemorrhage, Conscious Level (both adult and child) and Pain.* Specific discriminators are designed to ensure that patients with a significant mechanism of injury are given a high enough urgency, and that those with pre-existing medical conditions and or the development of new neurological signs are seen in good time

Specific discriminators	Explanation
Acutely short of breath	Shortness of breath that comes on suddenly, or a sudden exacerbation of chronic shortness of breath
Acute neurological deficit	Any loss of neurological function that has come on within the previous 24 hours. This might include altered or lost sensation, weakness of the limbs (either transiently or permanently) and alterations in bladder or bowel function
Significant mechanism of injury	Penetrating injuries (stab or gunshot) and injuries with high energy transfer such as falls from heights and high speed road traffic accidents (speed > 40 mph) are significant especially if there has been ejection from the vehicle, death(s) of other victim(s) of the accident or marked deformation of the vehicle
History of unconsciousness	There may be a reliable witness who can state whether the patient was unconscious (and for how long). If not a patient who is unable to remember the incident should be assumed to have been unconscious
Significant medical history	Any pre-existing medical condition requiring continual medication or other care

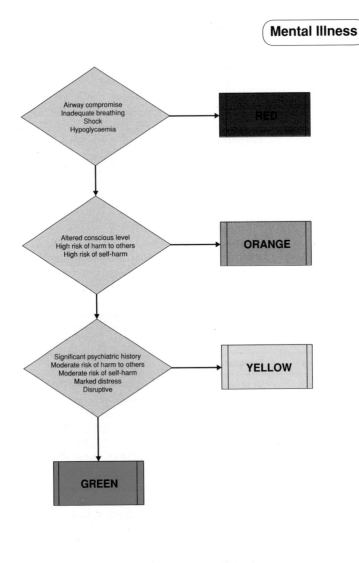

Mental Illness

Airway compromise
Inadequate breathing
Shock
Hypoglycaemia

→ RED

Altered conscious level
High risk of harm to others
High risk of self-harm

→ ORANGE

Significant psychiatric history
Moderate risk of harm to others
Moderate risk of self-harm
Marked distress
Disruptive

→ YELLOW

GREEN

R	O	Y	G	B
	Ma	Ma		

Notes Accompanying Mental Illness

See also	Chart notes
Behaving strangely Apparently drunk	This is a presentation defined flow diagram which has been designed to allow clinical prioritisation of patients who present with known or newly declared mental illness. This would include patients who attended with a chief complaint which would indicate mental illness. A number of general discriminators have been used including *Life Threat* and *Conscious Level.* This chart is designed to allow assessment of both physical and psychiatric aspects of the presentation Specific discriminators are included to allow accurate prioritisation of patients with a known significant psychiatric history and those who have varying degrees of risk of causing harm to others or to themselves. Patients who are disruptive or who are suffering severe distress are placed in the urgent category

Specific discriminators	Explanation
Hypoglycaemia	Glucose less than 3 mmol/l
High risk of harm to others	The presence of a potential risk of harm to others can be judged by looking at posture (tense and clenched), speech patterns (loud and using threatening words) and motor behaviour (restless, pacing). High risk should be assumed if weapons and potential victims are available, or if self control is lost
High risk of self-harm	An initial view of the risk of self-harm can be formed by considering the patients' behaviour. Patients who have a significant history of self-harm are actively trying to harm themselves or who are actively trying to leave with the intent of harming themselves are at high risk
Significant psychiatric history	A history of a major psychiatric illness or event
Moderate risk of harm to others	The presence of a potential risk of harm to others can be judged by looking at posture (tense and clenched), speech patterns (loud and using threatening words) and motor behaviour (restless, pacing). Moderate risk should be assumed if there is any indication of potential harm to others
Moderate risk of self-harm	An initial view of the risk of self-harm can be formed by considering the patients' behaviour. Patients without a significant history of self-harm, who are not actively trying to harm themselves, who are not actively trying to leave with the intent of harming themselves, but who profess the desire to harm themselves are at moderate risk
Marked distress	Patients who are markedly physically or emotionally upset fulfil this criterion
Disruptive	Disruptive behaviour is behaviour that affects the smooth running of the department. It may be threatening

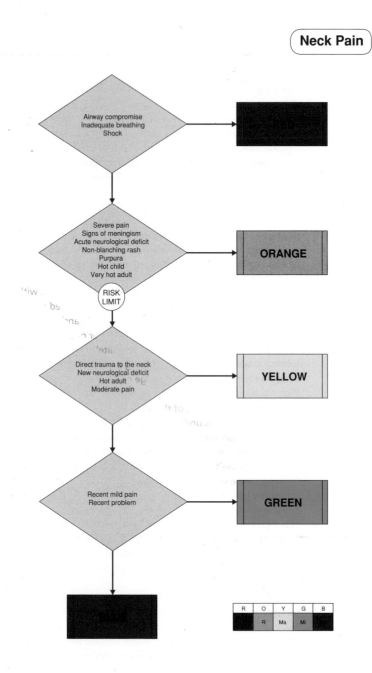

Neck Pain

Airway compromise
Inadequate breathing
Shock

Severe pain
Signs of meningism
Acute neurological deficit
Non-blanching rash
Purpura
Hot child
Very hot adult

ORANGE

RISK
LIMIT

Direct trauma to the neck
New neurological deficit
Hot adult
Moderate pain

YELLOW

Recent mild pain
Recent problem

GREEN

R	O	Y	G	B
	R	Ma	Mi	

Notes Accompanying Neck Pain

See also	Chart notes
Back pain Headache	This is a presentation defined flow diagram. Pain in the neck may arise because of local pathology or meningeal irritation. This chart is designed to allow rapid identification of patients presented with symptoms or signs which indicate more urgent pathologies. A number of general discriminators are used including *Life Threat, Pain and Temperature*. The specific discriminators which indicate meningitis are included under the ORANGE category

Specific discriminators	Explanation
Signs of meningism	Classically a stiff neck together with headache and photophobia
Acute neurological deficit	Any loss of neurological function that has come on within the previous 24 hours. This might include altered or lost sensation, weakness of the limbs (either transiently or permanently) and alterations in bladder or bowel function
Non-blanching rash	A rash that does not blanch (go white) when pressure is applied to it. Often tested using a glass tumbler to apply pressure as any colour change can be observed through the bottom of the tumbler
Purpura	A rash on any part of the body that is caused by small haemorrhages under the skin. A purpuric rash does not blanch (go white) when pressure is applied to it
Direct trauma to the neck	This may be top to bottom (loading) for instance when something falls on the head, bending (forwards, backwards or to the side), twisting or distracting such as in hanging
New neurological deficit	Any loss of neurological function including altered or lost sensation, weakness of the limbs (either transiently or permanently) and alterations in bladder or bowel function

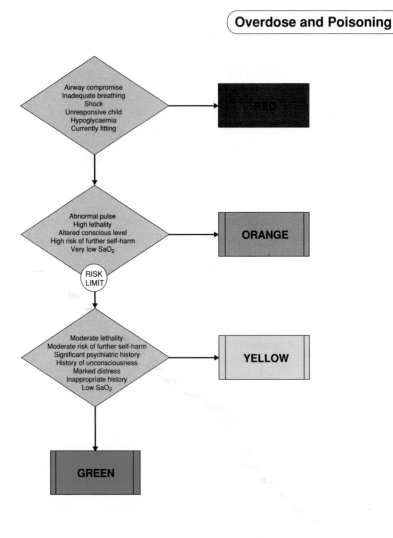

Overdose and Poisoning

Airway compromise
Inadequate breathing
Shock
Unresponsive child
Hypoglycaemia
Currently fitting

RED

Abnormal pulse
High lethality
Altered conscious level
High risk of further self-harm
Very low SaO$_2$

ORANGE

RISK LIMIT

Moderate lethality
Moderate risk of further self-harm
Significant psychiatric history
History of unconsciousness
Marked distress
Inappropriate history
Low SaO$_2$

YELLOW

GREEN

R	O	Y	G	B
	R	Ma		

Notes Accompanying Overdoses and Poisoning

See also	Chart notes
Deliberate self-harm	This is a presentation defined flow diagram. The flow chart has been designed to allow both the physical and psychiatric aspects of overdose to be considered, and to ensure accurate prioritisation of patients from both perspectives. It also allows prioritisation of patients who have been accidentally (or deliberately) poisoned by others
	A number of general discriminators have been used including *Life Threat and Unconscious Level (in both children and adults)*. Specific discriminators include the assessed lethality of the overdose (which can be decided following discussion with a Poisons Centre) and an assessment of the risk of further attempts at self-harm

Specific discriminators	Explanation
Hypoglycaemic	Glucose less than 3 mmol/l
Abnormal pulse	A bradycardia (<60 min in adults), a tachycardia (>100 min in adults) or an irregular rhythm. Age appropriate definitions of bradycardia and tachycardia should be used in children
High lethality	Lethality is the potential of the substance taken to cause harm. Advice from a Poisons Centre may be required to establish the level of risk of serious illness or death. If in doubt assume a high risk
High risk of further self-harm	An initial view of the risk of self-harm can be formed by considering the patients' behaviour Patients who have a significant history of self-harm, are actively trying to harm themselves or who are actively trying to leave with the intent of harming themselves are at high risk
Very low SaO$_2$	This is a saturation <95% on O$_2$ therapy or <90% on air
Moderate lethality	Lethality is the potential of the substance taken to cause serious illness or death. Advice from a Poisons Centre may be required to establish the level of risk to the patient
Moderate risk of further self-harm	An initial view of the risk of self-harm can be formed by considering the patients' behaviour. Patients without a significant history of self-harm, who are not actively trying to harm themselves, who are not actively trying to leave with the intent of harming themselves, but who profess the desire to harm themselves are at moderate risk
Significant psychiatric history	A history of a major psychiatric illness or event
History of unconsciousness	There may be a reliable witness who can state whether the patient was unconscious (and for how long). If not a patient who is unable to remember the incident should be assumed to have been unconscious
Marked distress	Patients who are markedly physically or emotionally upset fulfil this criterion
Inappropriate history	When the history (story) given does not explain the physical findings it is termed inappropriate. This is important as it is a marker of non-accidental injury in vulnerable children and adults and may be the sentinel for abuse
Low SaO$_2$	This is a saturation of <95% on air

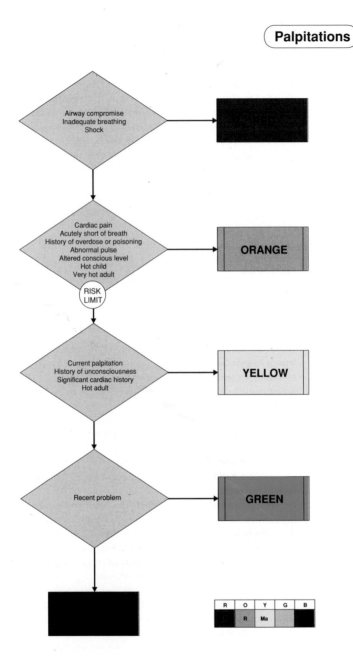

Notes Accompanying Palpitations

See also	Chart notes
Chest pain Unwell adult Collapsed adult	This is a presentation defined flow diagram designed to allow the accurate prioritisation of those patients that present with a chief complaint of palpitations
	Palpitations can have many causes ranging from the effects of ischaemic heart disease and other cardiac abnormalities to anxiety. Whatever the cause it is their effect on circulation and their propensity to develop into life-threatening dysrhythmias that determine the clinical priority of the patient. Thus this chart is written to ensure that the signs and symptoms of cardiac insufficiency are included in the RED and ORANGE categories, together with historical pointers to potential early problems

Specific discriminators	Explanation
Cardiac pain	Classically a severe dull 'gripping' or 'heavy' pain in the centre of the chest, radiating to the left arm or to the neck. May be associated with sweating and nausea
Acutely short of breath	Shortness of breath that comes on suddenly, or a sudden exacerbation of chronic shortness of breath
History of overdose and poisoning	This information may come from others or may be deduced if medication is missing
Abnormal pulse	A bradycardia (<60 min in adults), a tachycardia (>100 min in adults) or an irregular rhythm. Age appropriate definitions of bradycardia and tachycardia should be used in children
Current palpitation	A feeling of the heart racing (often described as a fluttering) that is still present
History of unconsciousness	There may be a reliable witness who can state whether the patient was unconscious (and for how long). If not a patient who is unable to remember the incident should be assumed to have been unconscious
Significant cardiac history	A known recurrent dysrhythmia which has life-threatening effects is significant as is a known cardiac condition that may deteriorate rapidly

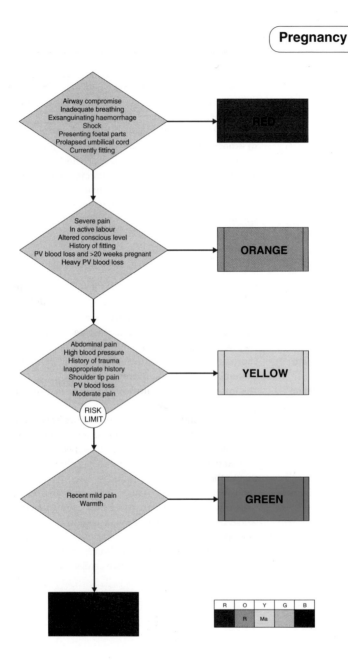

Pregnancy

Airway compromise
Inadequate breathing
Exsanguinating haemorrhage
Shock
Presenting foetal parts
Prolapsed umbilical cord
Currently fitting
→ RED

Severe pain
In active labour
Altered conscious level
History of fitting
PV blood loss and >20 weeks pregnant
Heavy PV blood loss
→ ORANGE

Abdominal pain
High blood pressure
History of trauma
Inappropriate history
Shoulder tip pain
PV blood loss
Moderate pain
→ YELLOW

RISK LIMIT

Recent mild pain
Warmth
→ GREEN

R	O	Y	G	B
	R	Ma		

Notes Accompanying Pregnancy

See also	Chart notes
PV bleeding	This is a presentation defined flow diagram. Pregnant women may attend the Emergency Department at all stages of pregnancy and with a variety of complaints. Some may be unaware of their pregnancy A number of general discriminators have been used including *Pain* and *Conscious Level*. Specific discriminators are designed to allow early recognition of complications of pregnancy at all stages

Specific discriminators	Explanation
Presenting foetal parts	Crowning or presentation of any other foetal part in the vagina
Prolapsed umbilical cord	Prolapse of any part of the umbilical cord through the cervix
In active labour	A woman who is having regular frequent painful contractions fulfils this criterion
History of fitting	Any observed or reported fits that have occurred during the period of illness or following an episode of trauma
PV blood loss and >20 weeks pregnant	Any loss of blood per vaginum in a woman known to be beyond the 20th week of pregnancy
Heavy PV blood loss	PV loss is extremely difficult to assess. The presence of large clots or constant flow fulfils this criterion. The use of a large number of sanitary towels is suggestive of heavy loss
High blood pressure	A history of raised blood pressure or a raised blood pressure on examination
History of trauma	A history of a recent physically traumatic event
Inappropriate history	When the history (story) given does not explain the physical findings it is termed inappropriate. This is important as it is a marker of non-accidental injury in vulnerable children and adults and may be the sentinel for abuse
Shoulder tip pain	Pain felt in the tip of the shoulder. This often indicates diaphragmatic irritation
PV blood loss	Any loss of blood per vaginum

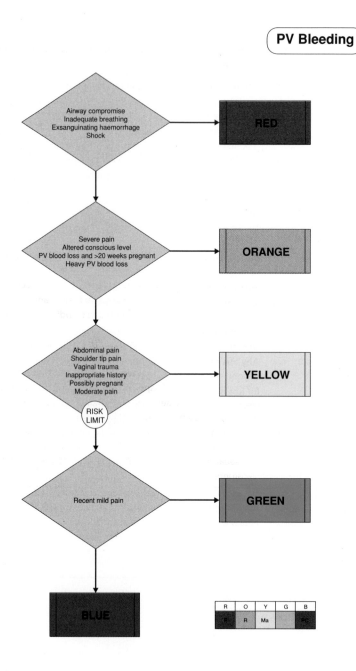

PV Bleeding

Airway compromise Inadequate breathing Exsanguinating haemorrhage Shock	**RED**

Severe pain Altered conscious level PV blood loss and >20 weeks pregnant Heavy PV blood loss	**ORANGE**

Abdominal pain Shoulder tip pain Vaginal trauma Inappropriate history Possibly pregnant Moderate pain	**YELLOW**

RISK LIMIT

Recent mild pain	**GREEN**

BLUE

R	O	Y	G	B
R	R	Ma		PC

Notes Accompanying PV Bleeding

See also	Chart notes
Pregnancy Abdominal pain	This is a presentation defined flow diagram. PV bleeding may occur in pregnant and non-pregnant women and may have a large number of undefined causes. A number of general discriminators are used including *Life Threat, Haemorrhage, and Pain*

Specific discriminators	Explanation
PV blood loss and >20 weeks pregnant	Any loss of blood per vaginum in a woman known to be beyond the 20th week of pregnancy
Heavy PV blood loss	PV loss is extremely difficult to assess. The presence of large clots or constant flow fulfils this criterion. The use of a large number of sanitary towels is suggestive of heavy loss
Abdominal pain	Any pain felt in the abdomen. Abdominal pain associated with back pain may indicate abdominal aortic aneurysm, whilst association with PV bleeding may indicate ectopic pregnancy or miscarriage
Shoulder tip pain	Pain felt in the tip of the shoulder. This often indicates diaphragmatic irritation
Inappropriate history	When the history (story) given does not explain the physical findings it is termed inappropriate. This is important as it is a marker of non-accidental injury in vulnerable children and adults and may be the sentinel for abuse
Possibly pregnant	Any woman whose normal menstruation has failed to occur is possibly pregnant. Furthermore any woman of childbearing age who is having unprotected sex should be considered to be potentially pregnant

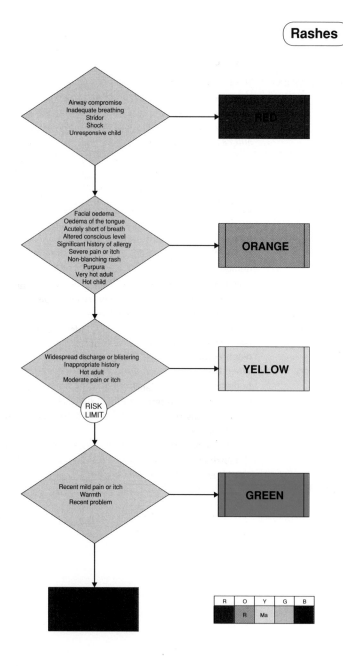

Rashes

Airway compromise
Inadequate breathing
Stridor
Shock
Unresponsive child

RED

Facial oedema
Oedema of the tongue
Acutely short of breath
Altered conscious level
Significant history of allergy
Severe pain or itch
Non-blanching rash
Purpura
Very hot adult
Hot child

ORANGE

Widespread discharge or blistering
Inappropriate history
Hot adult
Moderate pain or itch

YELLOW

RISK
LIMIT

Recent mild pain or itch
Warmth
Recent problem

GREEN

R	O	Y	G	B
	R	Ma		

Notes Accompanying Rashes

See also	Chart notes
Unwell child	This is a presentation defined flow diagram. A rash may
Unwell adult	signify serious disease such as meningococcal septicaemia, or
Allergy	may be a sign of a chronic non-acute problem such as
Bites and stings	psoriasis. Two general discriminators – *Life Threat and Temperature* – are used in this chart. A larger number of specific discriminators are included in the ORANGE and YELLOW categories to ensure that more *serious* conditions are suitably triaged. In particular purpura and associations of acute anaphylaxis appear at the ORANGE level

Specific discriminators	Explanation
Stridor	This may be an inspiratory or expiratory noise, or both. Stridor is heard best on breathing with the mouth open
Facial oedema	Diffuse swelling around the face usually involving the lips
Oedema of the tongue	Swelling of the tongue of any degree
Acutely short of breath	Shortness of breath that comes on suddenly, or a sudden exacerbation of chronic shortness of breath
Significant history of allergy	A known sensitivity with severe reaction (e.g. to nuts or bee sting) is significant
Non-blanching rash	A rash that does not blanch (go white) when pressure is applied to it. Often tested using a glass tumbler to apply pressure as any colour change can be observed through the bottom of the tumbler
Purpura	A rash on any part of the body that is caused by small haemorrhages under the skin. A purpuric rash does not blanch (go white) when pressure is applied to it
Widespread discharge or blistering	Any discharging or blistering eruption covering more than 10% body surface area

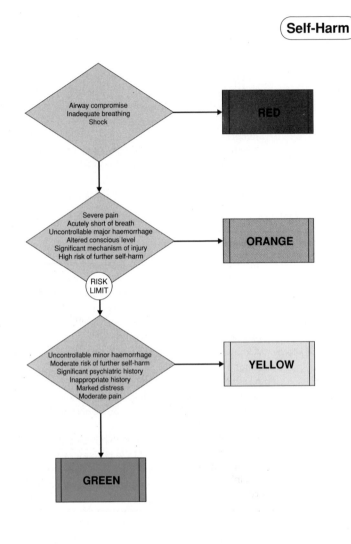

Self-Harm

RED

Airway compromise
Inadequate breathing
Shock

ORANGE

Severe pain
Acutely short of breath
Uncontrollable major haemorrhage
Altered conscious level
Significant mechanism of injury
High risk of further self-harm

RISK
LIMIT

YELLOW

Uncontrollable minor haemorrhage
Moderate risk of further self-harm
Significant psychiatric history
Inappropriate history
Marked distress
Moderate pain

GREEN

R	O	Y	G	B
R	R	Ma		

Notes Accompanying Self-Harm

See also	Chart notes
Overdose and poisoning Mental illness	This is a presentation defined flow diagram. This flow diagram has been designed to allow accurate prioritisation of patients who have caused physical harm to themselves. This chart is designed to allow assessment of both physical and psychiatric aspects of the presentation. A separate chart entitled overdoses and poisoning has been designed as well A number of general discriminators are used including *Life Threat, Haemorrhage, Conscious Level* and *Pain*. Specific discriminators are included to allow accurate prioritisation of patients with the significant mechanism of injury and those who have various degrees of risk of further self-harm

Specific discriminators	Explanation
Acutely short of breath	Shortness of breath that comes on suddenly, or a sudden exacerbation of chronic shortness of breath
Significant mechanism of injury	Penetrating injuries (stab or gunshot) and injuries with high energy transfer such as falls from heights and high speed road traffic accidents (speed >40 mph) are significant especially if there has been ejection from the vehicle, death(s) of other victim(s) of accident or marked deformation of the vehicle
High risk of further self-harm	An initial view of the risk of self-harm can be formed by considering the patients' behaviour. Patients who have a significant history of self-harm, are actively trying to harm themselves or who are actively trying to leave with the intent of harming themselves are at high risk
Moderate risk of further self-harm	An initial view of the risk of self-harm can be formed by considering the patients' behaviour. Patients without a significant history of self-harm, who are not actively trying to harm themselves, who are not actively trying to leave with the intent of harming themselves, but who profess the desire to harm themselves are at moderate risk
Significant psychiatric history	A history of a major psychiatric illness or event
Inappropriate history	When the history (story) given does not explain the physical findings it is termed inappropriate. This is important as it is a marker of non-accidental injury in vulnerable children and adults and may be the sentinel for abuse
Marked distress	Patients who are markedly physically or emotionally upset fulfil this criterion

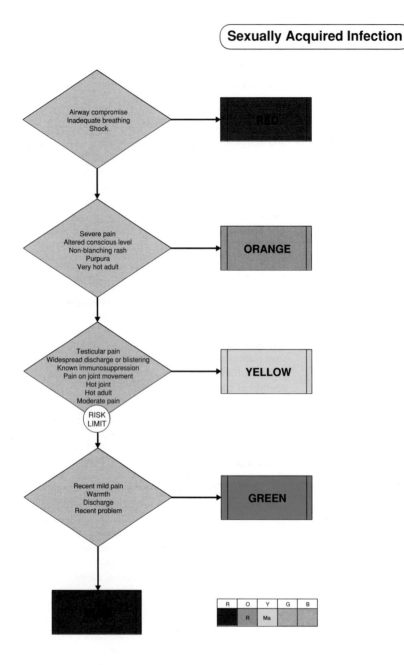

Notes Accompanying Sexually Acquired Infection

See also	Chart notes
	This is a presentation defined flow diagram which has been included to allow prioritisation of patients who attend with known or obvious sexual acquired infection. A number of general discriminators are used including *Life Threat, Pain and Temperature*. Specific discriminators have been added to allow identification of more urgent conditions such as gonococcocaemia
	It is important to ensure that preconceptions about disposal of these patients do not prevent appropriate triage

Specific discriminators	Explanation
Non-blanching rash	A rash that does not blanch (go white) when pressure is applied to it. Often tested using a glass tumbler to apply pressure as any colour change can be observed through the bottom of the tumbler
Purpura	A rash on any part of the body that is caused by small haemorrhages under the skin. A purpuric rash does not blanch (go white) when pressure is applied to it
Testicular pain	Pain in the testicles
Widespread discharge or blistering	Any discharging or blistering eruption covering more than 10% body surface area
Known immunosuppression	Any patient on immunosuppressive drugs (including long term steroids) or who is HIV positive
Pain on joint movement	This can be pain on either active (patient) movement or passive (examiner) movement
Discharge	In the context of sexually acquired infection this is any discharge from the penis or abnormal discharge from the vagina

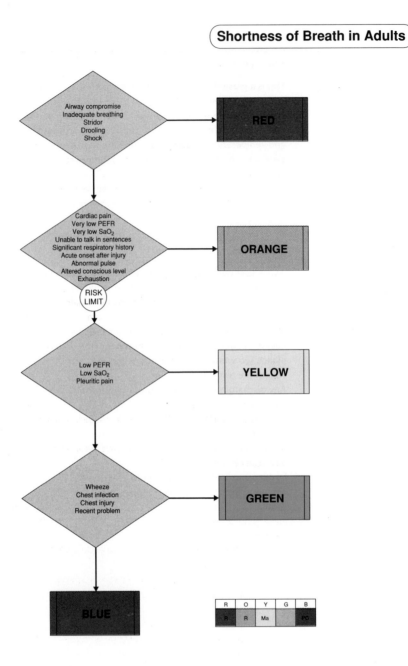

Shortness of Breath in Adults

Airway compromise
Inadequate breathing
Stridor
Drooling
Shock

RED

Cardiac pain
Very low PEFR
Very low SaO₂
Unable to talk in sentences
Significant respiratory history
Acute onset after injury
Abnormal pulse
Altered conscious level
Exhaustion

RISK LIMIT

ORANGE

Low PEFR
Low SaO₂
Pleuritic pain

YELLOW

Wheeze
Chest infection
Chest injury
Recent problem

GREEN

BLUE

R	O	Y	G	B
R	R	Ma		PC

Notes Accompanying Shortness of Breath in Adults

See also	Chart notes
Asthma Shortness of breath in children Unwell adult	This is a presentation defined flow diagram. Shortness of breath may be the presenting symptom for a number of cardiovascular and respiratory problems. A number of general discriminators are used including *Life Threat and Oxygen Saturation*. Specific discriminators include those which are present in severe asthma, chronic obstructive pulmonary disease and ischaemic heart disease

Specific discriminators	Explanation
Stridor	This may be an inspiratory or expiratory noise, or both. Stridor is heard best on breathing with the mouth open
Drooling	Saliva running from the mouth as a result of being unable to swallow
Cardiac pain	Classically a severe dull 'gripping' or 'heavy' pain in the centre of the chest, radiating to the left arm or to the neck. May be associated with sweating and nausea
Very low PEFR	This is a PEFR of 33% or less of best or predicted PEFR
Very low SaO_2	This is a saturation <95% on O_2 therapy or <90% on air
Unable to talk in sentences	Patients who are so breathless that they cannot complete relatively short sentences in one breath
Significant respiratory history	A history of previous life threatening episodes of a respiratory condition (e.g. COPD) is significant as is brittle asthma
Acute onset after injury	Onset of symptoms immediately within 24 hours of a physically traumatic event
Abnormal pulse	A bradycardia (<60 min in adults), a tachycardia (>100 min in adults) or an irregular rhythm
Exhaustion	Exhausted patients appear to reduce the effort they make to breathe despite continuing respiratory insufficiency. This is preterminal
Low PEFR	This is a PEFR of 50% or less of best or predicted PEFR
Low SaO_2	This is a saturation of <95% on air
Pleuritic pain	A sharp, localised pain in the chest that worsens on breathing, coughing or sneezing
Wheeze	This can be audible wheeze or a feeling of wheeze. Very severe airway obstruction is silent (no air can move)
Chest infection	A chest infection usually causes a cough and production of sputum. This is usually purulent (green or yellow)
Chest injury	Any injury to the area below the clavicles and above the level of the lowest rib. Injury to the lower part of the chest can cause underlying damage to abdominal organs

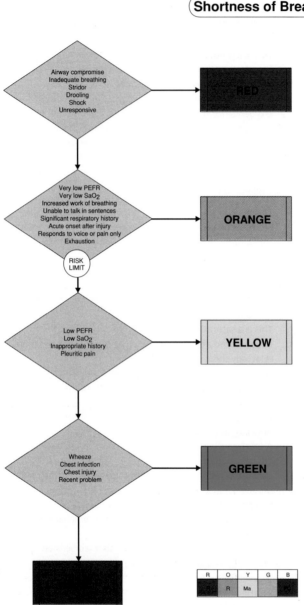

Shortness of Breath in Children

Airway compromise
Inadequate breathing
Stridor
Drooling
Shock
Unresponsive

RED

Very low PEFR
Very low SaO$_2$
Increased work of breathing
Unable to talk in sentences
Significant respiratory history
Acute onset after injury
Responds to voice or pain only
Exhaustion

RISK LIMIT

ORANGE

Low PEFR
Low SaO$_2$
Inappropriate history
Pleuritic pain

YELLOW

Wheeze
Chest infection
Chest injury
Recent problem

GREEN

R	O	Y	G	B
	R	Ma		

Notes Accompanying Shortness of Breath in Children

See also	Chart notes
Asthma Unwell child	This is a presentation defined flow diagram which applies to children under the age of 14. A number of general discriminators are used including *Life Threat and Oxygen Saturation*. Specific discriminators have been included to allow accurate identification of children who are suffering the severe effects of asthma and those in whom there is more serious pathology. Accurate peak flow reading is difficult in young children and in such cases this discriminator should be ignored. Peak flow readings when obtained should always be related to the expected peak flow for age and sex. The risk limit sits between ORANGE and YELLOW and therefore no children can be categorised as YELLOW, GREEN or BLUE until all the specific and general discriminators outlined under the RED and ORANGE categories have been specifically excluded. This may take longer than the time available for initial assessment

Specific discriminators	Explanation
Stridor	This may be an inspiratory or expiratory noise, or both. Stridor is heard best on breathing with the mouth open
Drooling	Saliva running from the mouth as a result of being unable to swallow
Very low PEFR	This is a PEFR of 33% or less of best or predicted PEFR
Very low SaO$_2$	This is a saturation <95% on O$_2$ therapy or <90% on air
Increased work of breathing	Increased work of breathing is shown as increased respiratory rate, use of accessory muscles and grunting
Unable to talk in sentences	Patients who are so breathless that they cannot complete relatively short sentences in one breath
Significant respiratory history	A history of previous life threatening episodes of a respiratory condition is significant as is brittle asthma
Acute onset after injury	Onset of symptoms immediately within 24 hours of a physically traumatic event
Exhaustion	An exhausted patient appears to reduce the effort they make to breathe despite continuing respiratory insufficiency. This is preterminal
Low PEFR	This is a PEFR of 50% or less of best or predicted PEFR
Low SaO$_2$	This is a saturation of <95% on air
Inappropriate history	When the history (story) given does not explain the physical findings it is termed inappropriate. This is important as it is a marker of non-accidental injury in vulnerable children and adults and may be the sentinel for abuse
Pleuritic pin	A sharp, localised pain in the chest that worsens on breathing, coughing or sneezing
Wheeze	This can be audible wheeze or a feeling of wheeze. Very severe airway obstruction is silent (no air can move)
Chest infection	A chest infection usually causes a cough and production of sputum. This is usually purulent (green or yellow)
Chest injury	Any injury to the area below the clavicles and above the level of the lowest rib. Injury to the lower part of the chest can cause underlying damage to abdominal organs

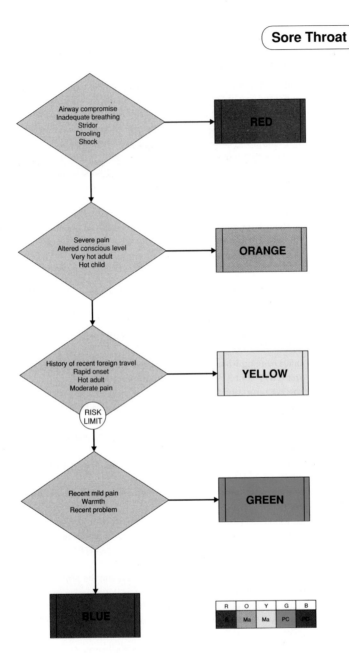

Sore Throat

Airway compromise
Inadequate breathing
Stridor
Drooling
Shock

RED

Severe pain
Altered conscious level
Very hot adult
Hot child

ORANGE

History of recent foreign travel
Rapid onset
Hot adult
Moderate pain

YELLOW

RISK LIMIT

Recent mild pain
Warmth
Recent problem

GREEN

BLUE

R	O	Y	G	B
R	Ma	Ma	PC	PC

Notes Accompanying Sore Throat

See also	Chart notes
Unwell adult Unwell child Shortness of breath in adults Shortness of breath in children	This is a presentation defined flow diagram designed to allow accurate prioritisation for patients attending with sore throat. As problems with the throat can affect the air way there are a number of conditions which have this presentation and have a high priority. A number of general discriminators are used including *Life Threat, Pain and Temperature*. Specific discriminators have been included to indicate high chance of more serious pathology

Specific discriminators	Explanation
Stridor	This may be an inspiratory or expiratory noise, or both. Stridor is heard best on breathing with the mouth open
Drooling	Saliva running from the mouth as a result of being unable to swallow
History of foreign travel	Recent foreign travel (within 2 weeks)
Rapid onset	Onset within the preceding 12 hours

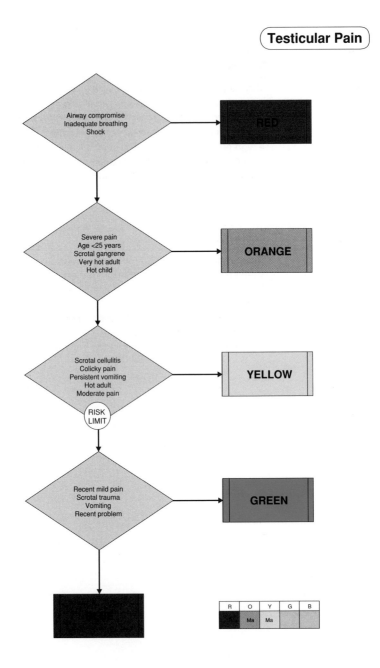

Testicular Pain

Airway compromise
Inadequate breathing
Shock

RED

Severe pain
Age <25 years
Scrotal gangrene
Very hot adult
Hot child

ORANGE

Scrotal cellulitis
Colicky pain
Persistent vomiting
Hot adult
Moderate pain

RISK
LIMIT

YELLOW

Recent mild pain
Scrotal trauma
Vomiting
Recent problem

GREEN

R	O	Y	G	B
	Ma	Ma		

Notes Accompanying Testicular Pain

See also	Chart notes
Abdominal pain	This is a presentation defined flow diagram. Testicular pain may have a number of pathologies the most urgent of which is testicular torsion. A number of general discriminators are used including *Life Threat, Pain and Temperature*. Specific discriminators included in the ORANGE category are designed to indicate those patients who have a high chance or torsion of the testes and the most severe infections

Specific discriminators	Explanation
Age <25 years	25 years old or younger
Scrotal gangrene	Dead blackened skin around the scrotum and groin. Early gangrene may not be black but may appear like a full thickness burn with or without flaking
Scrotal cellulitis	Redness and swelling around the scrotum
Colicky pain	Pain that comes and goes in waves. Renal colic tends to come and go over 20 minutes or so
Persistent vomiting	Vomiting that is continuous or that occurs without any respite between episodes
Scrotal trauma	Any recent physically traumatic event involving the scrotum

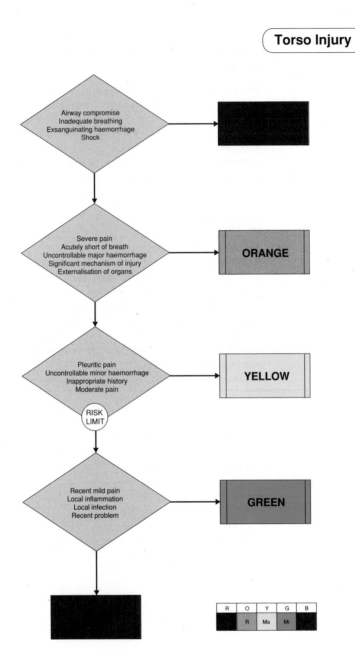

Torso Injury

Airway compromise
Inadequate breathing
Exsanguinating haemorrhage
Shock

RED

Severe pain
Acutely short of breath
Uncontrollable major haemorrhage
Significant mechanism of injury
Externalisation of organs

ORANGE

Pleuritic pain
Uncontrollable minor haemorrhage
Inappropriate history
Moderate pain

YELLOW

RISK
LIMIT

Recent mild pain
Local inflammation
Local infection
Recent problem

GREEN

BLUE

Notes Accompanying Torso Injury

See also	Chart notes
Major trauma Assault Wounds	This is a presentation defined flow diagram designed to allow accurate prioritisation of patients who have suffered injuries to the front or back of the chest and abdomen. A number of general discriminators are used including *Life Threat, Haemorrhage and Pain* Specific discriminators have been used to allow identification of patients who are suffering from less obvious but severe internal injury. These would include patients who are acutely short of breath and those with a history suggestive of significant trauma

Specific discriminators	Explanation
Acutely short of breath	Shortness of breath that comes on suddenly, or a sudden exacerbation of chronic shortness of breath
Significant mechanism of injury	Penetrating injuries (stab or gunshot) and injuries with high energy transfer such as falls from heights and high speed road traffic accidents (speed >40 mph) are significant especially if there has been ejection from the vehicle, death(s) of other victim(s) of the accident or marked deformation of the vehicle
Pleuritic pain	A sharp, localised pain in the chest that worsens on breathing, coughing or sneezing
Inappropriate history	When the history (story) given does not explain the physical findings it is termed inappropriate. This is important as it is a marker of non-accidental injury in vulnerable children and adults and may be the sentinel for abuse
Local inflammation	Local inflammation will involve pain, swelling and redness confined to a particular site or area
Local infection	Local infection usually manifests as inflammation (pain, swelling and redness) confined to a particular site or area, with or without a collection of pus

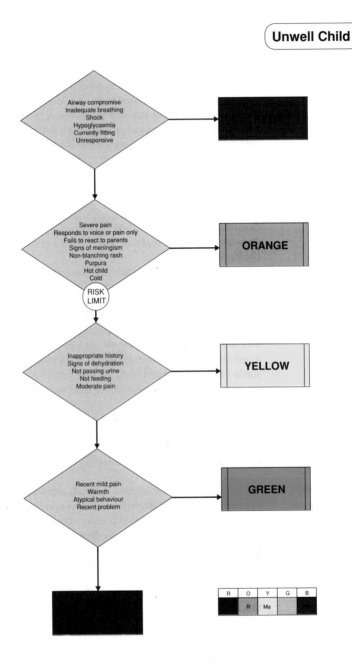

Notes Accompanying Torso Injury

See also	Chart notes
Major trauma Assault Wounds	This is a presentation defined flow diagram designed to allow accurate prioritisation of patients who have suffered injuries to the front or back of the chest and abdomen. A number of general discriminators are used including *Life Threat, Haemorrhage and Pain* Specific discriminators have been used to allow identification of patients who are suffering from less obvious but severe internal injury. These would include patients who are acutely short of breath and those with a history suggestive of significant trauma

Specific discriminators	Explanation
Acutely short of breath	Shortness of breath that comes on suddenly, or a sudden exacerbation of chronic shortness of breath
Significant mechanism of injury	Penetrating injuries (stab or gunshot) and injuries with high energy transfer such as falls from heights and high speed road traffic accidents (speed >40 mph) are significant especially if there has been ejection from the vehicle, death(s) of other victim(s) of the accident or marked deformation of the vehicle
Pleuritic pain	A sharp, localised pain in the chest that worsens on breathing, coughing or sneezing
Inappropriate history	When the history (story) given does not explain the physical findings it is termed inappropriate. This is important as it is a marker of non-accidental injury in vulnerable children and adults and may be the sentinel for abuse
Local inflammation	Local inflammation will involve pain, swelling and redness confined to a particular site or area
Local infection	Local infection usually manifests as inflammation (pain, swelling and redness) confined to a particular site or area, with or without a collection of pus

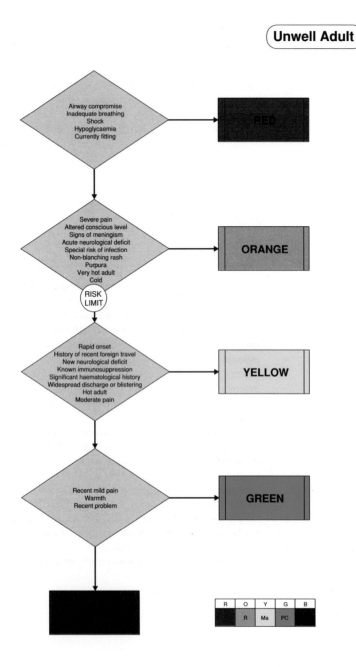

Unwell Adult

Airway compromise
Inadequate breathing
Shock
Hypoglycaemia
Currently fitting

RED

Severe pain
Altered conscious level
Signs of meningism
Acute neurological deficit
Special risk of infection
Non-blanching rash
Purpura
Very hot adult
Cold

RISK LIMIT

ORANGE

Rapid onset
History of recent foreign travel
New neurological deficit
Known immunosuppression
Significant haematological history
Widespread discharge or blistering
Hot adult
Moderate pain

YELLOW

Recent mild pain
Warmth
Recent problem

GREEN

R	O	Y	G	B
	R	Ma	PC	

Notes Accompanying Unwell Adult

See also	Chart notes
Collapsed adult	This is a non-specific presentation defined flow diagram. A number of general discriminators are used including *Life Threat, Conscious Level, Pain and Temperature.* Specific discriminators have been included to ensure that patients with, for example, meningococcocaemia are placed in the appropriate category

Specific discriminators	Explanation
Hypoglycaemia	Glucose less than 3 mmol/l
Signs of meningism	Classically a stiff neck together with headache and photophobia
Acute neurological deficit	Any loss of neurological function that has come on within the previous 24 hours. This might include altered or lost sensation, weakness of the limbs (either transiently or permanently) and alterations in bladder or bowel function
Special risk of infection	Known exposure to a dangerous pathogen, or travel to an area with an identified, current serious infectious risk
Non-blanching rash	A rash that does not blanch (go white) when pressure is applied to it. Often tested using a glass tumbler to apply pressure as any colour change can be observed through the bottom of the tumbler
Purpura	A rash on any part of the body that is caused by small haemorrhages under the skin. A purpuric rash does not blanch (go white) when pressure is applied to it
History of recent foreign travel	Recent foreign travel (within 2 weeks)
New neurological deficit	Any loss of neurological function including altered or lost sensation, weakness of the limbs (either transiently or permanently) and alterations in bladder or bowel function
Known immunosuppression	Any patient on immunosuppressive drugs (including long term steroids) or who is HIV positive
Significant haematological history	A patient with a haematological disorder that is known to deteriorate rapidly
Widespread discharge or blistering	Any discharging or blistering eruption covering more than 10% body surface area

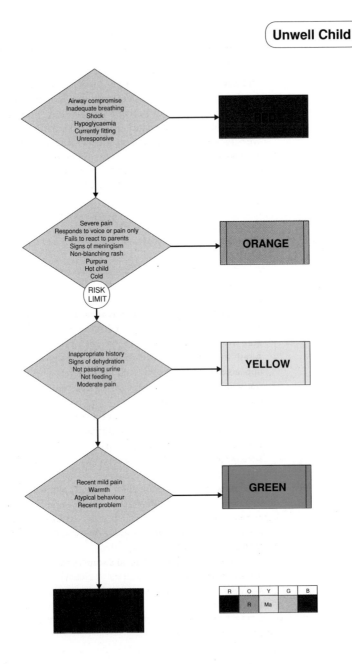

Unwell Child

Airway compromise
Inadequate breathing
Shock
Hypoglycaemia
Currently fitting
Unresponsive

RED

Severe pain
Responds to voice or pain only
Fails to react to parents
Signs of meningism
Non-blanching rash
Purpura
Hot child
Cold

RISK LIMIT

ORANGE

Inappropriate history
Signs of dehydration
Not passing urine
Not feeding
Moderate pain

YELLOW

Recent mild pain
Warmth
Atypical behaviour
Recent problem

GREEN

R	O	Y	G	B
	R	Ma		

Notes Accompanying Unwell Child

See also	Chart notes
Crying baby Irritable child Worried parent	This is a presentation defined flow diagram designed to allow accurate prioritisation of children who present with non-specific illness. A number of general discriminators are used including *Life Threat, Conscious Level, Pain and Temperature*. A number of specific discriminators have been included to allow identification of more serious pathology such as meningoacoccocaemia, etc. The risk limit sits between ORANGE and YELLOW and therefore no children can be categorised as YELLOW, GREEN or BLUE until all the specific and general discriminators outlined under the RED and ORANGE categories have been specifically excluded. This may take longer than the time available for initial assessment

Specific discriminators	Explanation
Hypoglycaemia	Glucose less than 3 mmol/l
Fails to react to parents	Failure to react in any way to a parent's face or voice. Abnormal reactions and apparent lack of recognition of a parent are also worrying signs
Signs of meningism	Classically a stiff neck together with headache and photophobia
Non-blanching rash	A rash that does not blanch (go white) when pressure is applied to it. Often tested using a glass tumbler to apply pressure as any colour change can be observed through the bottom of the tumbler
Purpura	A rash on any part of the body that is caused by small haemorrhages under the skin. A purpuric rash does not blanch (go white) when pressure is applied to it
Inappropriate history	When the history (story) given does not explain the physical findings it is termed inappropriate. This is important as it is a marker of non-accidental injury in vulnerable children and adults and may be the sentinel for abuse
Signs of dehydration	These include dry tongue, sunken eyes, increased skin turgor and, in small babies, a sunken anterior fontanelle. Usually associated with a low urine output
Not passing urine	Failure to produce and pass urine. This may be difficult to judge in children and reference to the number of nappies or pads used may be useful
Not feeding	Children who will not take any solid or liquid (as appropriate) by mouth. Children who will take the food but always vomit afterwards may also fulfil this criterion
Atypical behaviour	Children who are behaving in a way that is not usual in the given situation. The carers will often volunteer this information. Such children are often referred to as fractious or 'out of sorts'

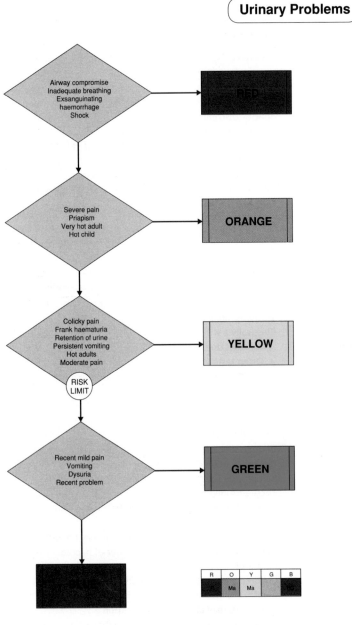

Urinary Problems

Notes Accompanying Urinary Problems

See also	Chart notes
Sexually acquired infection Testicular pain	This is a presentation defined flow diagram. A lot of patients who present with urinary problems are in pain and some may have serious underlying pathology. A number of general discriminators are used including life threat, pain and temperature. Specific discriminators have been included to ensure that patients suffering from urinary retention and those with infections are included in the appropriate categories

Specific discriminators	Explanation
Priapism	Sustained penile erection
Colicky pain	Pain that comes and goes in waves. Renal colic tends to come and go over 20 min or so
Frank haematuria	Red discolouration of the urine caused by blood
Retention of urine	Inability to pass urine per urethra associated with an enlarged bladder. This condition is usually very painful unless there is altered sensation
Persistent vomiting	Vomiting that is continuous or that occurs without any respite between episodes
Dysuria	Pain or difficulty in passing urine. Pain is typically described as stinging or hot

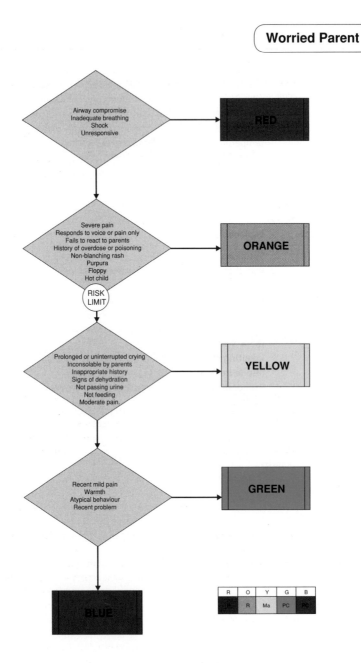

Notes Accompanying Worried Parent

See also	Chart notes

Crying baby
Irritable child
Unwell child
	This is a presentation defined flow diagram which has been designed to allow accurate prioritisation of children who are brought to the attention of the service because of parental worry. Parents know their children better than anyone else and although many of these children will not have serious pathology it is essential that these presentations are taken seriously
	    A number of general discriminators are used including *Life Threat, Conscious Level, Pain and Temperature*. Specific discriminators have been added to the chart to allow identification of more serious pathologies which are apparent or may potentially exist
	    The risk limit sits between ORANGE and YELLOW and therefore no children can be categorised as YELLOW, GREEN or BLUE until all the specific and general discriminators outlined under the RED and ORANGE categories have been specifically excluded. This may take longer than the time available for initial assessment

Specific discriminators	Explanation
Fails to react to parents	Failure to react in any way to a parent's face or voice. Abnormal reactions and apparent lack of recognition of a parent are also worrying signs
History of overdose or poisoning	This information may come from others or may be deduced if medication is missing
Non-blanching rash	A rash that does not blanch (go white) when pressure is applied to it. Often tested using a glass tumbler to apply pressure as any colour change can be observed through the bottom of the tumbler
Purpura	A rash on any part of the body that is caused by small haemorrhages under the skin. A purpuric rash does not blanch (go white) when pressure is applied to it
Floppy	Parents may describe their children as floppy. Tone is generally reduced – the most noticeable sign is often lolling of the head
Prolonged or uninterrupted crying	A child who has cried continuously for 2 hours or more fulfils this criterion
Inconsolable by parents	Children whose crying or distress does not respond to attempts by their parents to comfort them fulfil this criterion
Inappropriate history	When the history (story) given does not explain the physical findings it is termed inappropriate. This is important as it is a marker of non-accidental injury in vulnerable children and adults and may be the sentinel for abuse
Signs of dehydration	These include dry tongue, sunken eyes, increased skin turgor and, in small babies, a sunken anterior fontanelle. Usually associated with a low urine output
Not passing urine	Failure to produce and pass urine. This may be difficult to judge in children and reference to the number of nappies or pads used may be useful
Not feeding	Children who will not take any solid or liquid (as appropriate) by mouth. Children who will take the food but always vomit afterwards may also fulfil this criterion
Atypical behaviour	Children who are behaving in a way that is not usual in the given situation. The carers will often volunteer this information. Such children are often referred to as fractious or 'out of sorts'

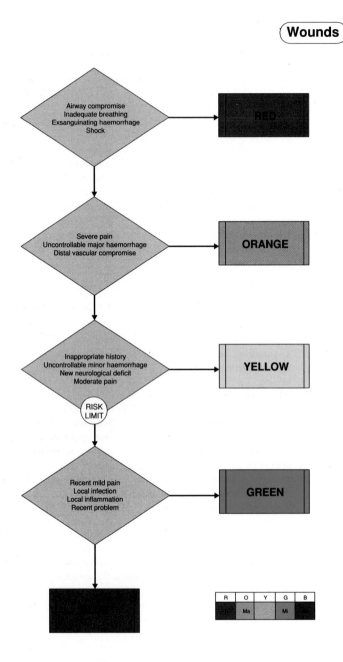

Notes Accompanying Wounds

See also	Chart notes
Assault	This is a presentation defined flow diagram. Many patients attend all forms of emergency care suffering from wounds of various nature. These vary from severe life threatening lacerations to minor abrasions. This chart is designed to allow an accurate prioritisation of these patients A number of general discriminators have been used including *Life Threat, Haemorrhage and Pain*. Specific discriminators have been included to allow identification of patients with signs and symptoms suggesting injuries which pose a threat to function

Specific discriminators	Explanation
Distal vascular compromise	There will be a combination of pallor, coldness, altered sensation and pain with or without absent pulses distal to the injury
Inappropriate history	When the history (story) given does not explain the physical findings it is termed inappropriate. This is important as it is a marker of non-accidental injury in vulnerable children and adults and may be the sentinel for abuse
New neurological deficit	Any loss of neurological function including altered or lost sensation, weakness of the limbs (either transiently or permanently) and alterations in bladder or bowel function
Local infection	Local infection usually manifests as inflammation (pain, swelling and redness) confined to a particular site or area, with or without a collection of pus
Local inflammation	Local inflammation will involve pain, swelling and redness confined to a particular site or area

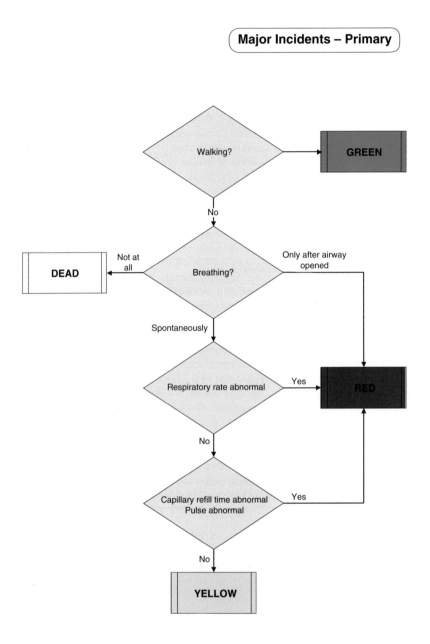

Notes Accompanying Major Incidents – Primary

See also	Chart notes
Major incidents – secondary	Triage during a major incident has a completely different aim from that during the day to day running of emergency services. To achieve this aim (which is to initially save as many lives as possible and then to deliver the best care possible within the existing resources) a different approach has been taken. Rather than select the most seriously ill first in this instance the least ill are selected. Rather than using general and specific discriminators, very broad brush discriminators are used which allow rough division of patients into three categories
	This chart describes the first 'sorting' triage method for use in major incidents. It is designed to allow rapid imposition of order when a large number of untriaged casualties arrive at once. It does not pick out the most severe first, rather selecting the most numerous (walking) and then subcategorising the stretcher patients as dead, red or yellow. Inevitably this quick method is not totally accurate, and other methods should be used once time allows
	No longer than 15 seconds should be spent on each patient

Specific discriminators	Explanation
Walking	The ability to walk (whatever the injury) is used as a discriminator to select patient of the standard category
Breathing after airway opened	Patients who cannot breathe after their airway is opened are considered dead unless considerable life support resources exist
Respiratory rate abnormal	Casualties whose respiratory rate is abnormal either by being too high (over 29) or too low (less than 10) are categorised as RED
Capillary refill time abnormal	Casualties whose capillary refill is prolonged (more than 2 seconds) are categorised as RED
Pulse rate abnormal	If the capillary refill time cannot be measured then casualties whose pulse is raised over 120 beats per minute are categorised RED
	All other patients are placed in the YELLOW category

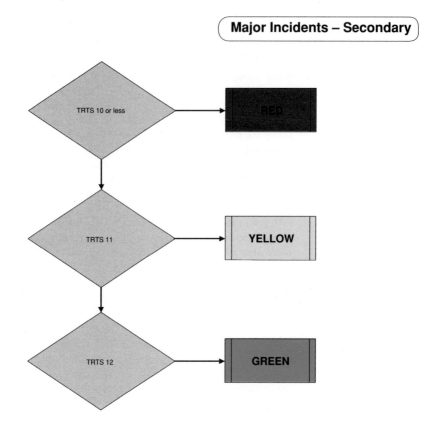

Notes Accompanying Major Incidents – Secondary

See also	Chart notes

Major incidents – primary	The primary major incident triage methodology is used to rapidly screen a large number of patients into broad brush categories.
	The Triage Revised Trauma Score (TRTS) is a slightly more refined physiological approach to the triage of a large number of casualties. It is based on the coded values of three physiological parameters
	Priorities are allocated from the TRTS as follows:
	    1–10 Priority 1
	    11 Priority 2
	    12 Priority 3
	    (0 Priority 4)

Specific discriminators	Explanation
TRTS	Triage revised trauma score
Respiratory rate	
10–29	4
>29	3
6–9	2
1–5	1
0	0
Systolic blood pressure	
90	4
76–89	3
50–75	2
1–49	1
0	0
Glasgow Coma Scale score	
13–15	4
9–12	3
6–8	2
4–5	1
3	0

Discriminator dictionary

Abdominal pain	Any pain felt in the abdomen. Abdominal pain associated with back pain may indicate abdominal aortic aneurysm, whilst association with PV bleeding may indicate ectopic pregnancy or miscarriage
Abnormal pulse	A bradycardia (<60 min in adults), a tachycardia (>100 min in adults) or an irregular rhythm. Age appropriate definitions of bradycardia and tachycardia should be used in children
Abrupt onset	Onset within seconds or minutes. May cause waking in sleep
Acute chemical eye injury	Any substance splashed into or placed into the eye within the past 24 hours that caused stinging, burning, or reduced vision should be assumed to have caused chemical injury
Acute complete loss of vision	Loss of vision in one or both eyes within the preceding 24 hours which has not returned to normal
Acute neurological deficit	Any loss of neurological function that has come on within the previous 24 hours. This might include altered or lost sensation, weakness of the limbs (either transiently or permanently) and alterations in bladder or bowel function
Acute onset after injury	Onset of symptoms immediately within 24 hours of a physically traumatic event
Acutely avulsed tooth	A tooth that has been avulsed intact within the previous 24 hours
Acutely short of breath	Shortness of breath that comes on suddenly, or a sudden exacerbation of chronic shortness of breath
Age less than 25 years	25 years old or younger
Airway compromise	An airway may be compromised either because it cannot be kept open or because the airway protective reflexes (that stop inhalation) have been lost. Failure to keep the airway open will result either in intermittent total obstruction or in partial obstruction. This will manifest itself as snoring or bubbling sounds during breathing

Altered blood	Darker than fresh blood and often smelling more like melaena
Altered conscious level	Not fully alert. Either responding to voice or pain only or unresponsive
Altered conscious level not wholly attributable to alcohol	A patient who is not fully alert, with a history of alcohol ingestion and in whom there is no doubt at all that other causes of reduced conscious level may be present fulfils this discriminator definition
Altered conscious level wholly attributable to alcohol	A patient who is not fully alert, with a clear history of alcohol ingestion and in whom there is no doubt that all other causes of reduced conscious level have been excluded fulfils this discriminator definition
Altered facial sensation	Any alteration of sensation on the face
Atypical behaviour	Children who are behaving in a way that is not usual in the given situation. The carers will often volunteer this information. Such children are often referred to as fractious or 'out of sorts'
Auricular haematoma	A tense haematoma (usually post traumatic) in the outer ear
Black stool	Any blackness fulfils this criterion
Bleeding disorder	Congenital or acquired bleeding disorder
Breathing after airway opened	In major incidents the presence of breathing after simple airway opening manoeuvres allows respiratory rate to be counted. Absence of breathing when the airway is open indicates death
Capillary refill time	The capillary refill time is the time taken for the nail bed capillaries to refill after pressure has been applied for 5 seconds. The normal time is less than 2 seconds. This sign is less useful if the patient is cold
Capillary refill time abnormal	Major incident casualties whose capillary refill is prolonged (more than 2 seconds) are categorised as RED
Cardiac pain	Classically a severe dull 'gripping' or 'heavy' pain in the centre of the chest, radiating to the left arm or to the neck. May be associated with sweating and nausea
Chemical injury	Any substance splashed onto or placed onto the body that causes stinging, burning, reduced vision or any other symptoms should be assumed to be capable of causing a chemical injury

Chest infection	A chest infection usually causes a cough and production of sputum. This is usually purulent (green or yellow)
Chest injury	Any injury to the area below the clavicles and above the level of the lowest rib. Injury to the lower part of the chest can cause underlying damage to abdominal organs
Cold	If the skin feels cold the patient is clinically said to be cold. The temperature should be taken as soon as possible – a core temperature $<35°C$ is cold
Colicky pain	Pain that comes and goes in waves. Renal colic tends to come and go over 20 min or so
Critical skin	A fracture or dislocation may leave fragments or ends of bone pressing so hard against the skin that the viability of the skin is threatened. The skin will be white and under tension
Currently fitting	Patients who are in the tonic or clonic stages of a grand mal convulsion, and patients currently experiencing partial fits fulfil this criterion
Current palpitation	A feeling of the heart racing (often described as a fluttering) that is still present
Deformity	This will always be subjective. Abnormal angulation or rotation is implied
Diplopia	Double vision which resolves when one eye is closed
Direct trauma to the back	This may be top to bottom (loading) for instance when people fall and land on their feet, bending (forwards, backwards or to the side) or twisting
Direct trauma to the neck	This may be top to bottom (loading) for instance when something falls on the head, bending (forwards, backwards or to the side), twisting or distracting such as in hanging
Discharge	In the context of sexually acquired infection this is any discharge from the penis or abnormal discharge from the vagina
Disruptive	Disruptive behaviour is behaviour that affects the smooth running of the department. It may be threatening
Distal vascular compromise	There will be a combination of pallor, coldness, altered sensation and pain with or without absent pulses distal to the injury

Distressed by pain	A child who is distressed by pain and inconsolable
Drooling	Saliva running from the mouth as a result of being unable to swallow
Dysuria	Pain or difficulty in passing urine. Pain is typically described as stinging or hot
Electrical injury	Any injury caused or possibly caused by electric current. This includes AC and DC and both artificial and natural sources
Exhaustion	Exhausted patients appear to reduce the effort they make to breathe despite continuing respiratory insufficiency. This is preterminal
Exsanguinating haemorrhage	Haemorrhage which is occurring at such a rate that death will ensue unless bleeding is stopped
Externalisation of organs	Herniation or frank extrusion of internal organs
Eye injury	A recent physically traumatic event to the eye
Facial oedema	Diffuse swelling around the face usually involving the lips
Facial swelling	Swelling around the face which may be localised or diffuse
Fails to react to parents	Failure to react in any way to a parent's face or voice. Abnormal reactions and apparent lack of recognition of a parent are also worrying signs
Floppy	Parents may describe their children as floppy. Tone is generally reduced – the most noticeable sign is often lolling of the head
Focal or progressive loss of function	Loss of function that is limited to a particular part of the body (limb, side, eye, etc.) or a loss of function that is getting worse over hours
Foreign body sensation	A sensation of something in the eye, often expressed as scraping or grittiness
Frank haematuria	Red discolouration of the urine caused by blood
Fresh blood	Unaltered blood – readily identified by both the patient and their carers
Generalised rash	The rash may be of any form but will usually be erythematous or urticarial
Gross deformity	This will always be subjective. Gross and abnormal angulation or rotation is implied
Headache	Any pain around the head that is not related to a particular anatomical structure. Facial pain is not included

Head injury	Any traumatic event involving the head fulfils this criterion
Heavy PV blood loss	PV loss is extremely difficult to assess. The presence of large clots or constant flow fulfils this criterion. The use of a large number of sanitary towels is suggestive of heavy loss
High blood pressure	A history of raised blood pressure or a raised blood pressure on examination
High lethality	Lethality is the potential of the substance taken to cause harm. Advice from a Poisons Centre may be required to establish the level of risk of serious illness or death. If in doubt assume a high risk
High lethality envenomation	Lethality is the potential of the envenomation to cause harm. Local knowledge may allow identification of the venomous creature, but advice may be required. If in doubt assume a high risk
High risk of (further) harm to others	The presence of a potential risk of harm to others can be judged by looking at posture (tense and clenched) speech patterns (loud and using threatening words) and motor behaviour (restless, pacing). High risk should be assumed if weapons and potential victims are available, or if self control is lost
High risk of (further) self-harm	An initial view of the risk of self-harm can be formed by considering the patients' behaviour. Patients who have a significant history of self-harm, are actively trying to harm themselves or who are actively trying to leave with the intent of harming themselves are at high risk
History of acutely vomiting blood	Frank haematemesis, vomiting of altered blood (coffee ground) or of blood mixed in the vomit within the past 24 hours
History of fitting	Any observed or reported fits that have occurred during the period of illness or following and episode of trauma
History of head injury	A history of a recent physically traumatic event involving the head. Usually this will be reported by the patient but if the patient has been unconscious this history should be sought from a reliable witness
History of overdose or poisoning	This information may come from others or may be deduced if medication is missing

History of recent foreign travel	Recent foreign travel (within 2 weeks)
History of trauma	A history of a recent physically traumatic event
History of unconsciousness	There may be a reliable witness who can state whether the patient was unconscious (and for how long). If not a patient who is unable to remember the incident should be assumed to have been unconscious
Hot adult	A temperature >38.5°C is hot
Hot child	If the skin feels hot the child is clinically said to be hot. The temperature should be taken as soon as possible – a temperature >38.5°C is hot
Hot joint	Any warmth around a joint fulfils this criterion. Often accompanied by redness
Hyperglycaemic	Glucose greater than 17 mmol/l
Hyperglycaemic with ketosis	Glucose greater than 11 mmol/l with urinary ketones or signs of acidosis (deep sighing respiration, etc.)
Hypoglycaemic	Glucose less than 3 mmol/l
Inability to bear weight	Inability to carry the full weight of the body through one or both lower limbs. This may be because of pain or loss of function
In active labour	A woman who is having regular and frequent painful contractions fulfils this criterion
Inadequate breathing	Patients who are failing to breathe well enough to maintain adequate oxygenation have inadequate breathing. There may be an increased work of breathing, signs of inadequate breathing or exhaustion
Inadequate history	If there is no clear and unequivocal history of acute alcohol ingestion, and if head injury, drug ingestion, underlying medical condition, etc. cannot be definitely excluded then the history is inadequate
Inappropriate history	When the history (story) given does not explain the physical findings it is termed inappropriate. This is important as it is a marker of non-accidental injury in vulnerable children and adults and may be the sentinel for abuse
Inconsolable by parents	Children whose crying or distress does not respond to attempts by their parents to comfort them fulfil this criterion

Increased work of breathing	Increased work of breathing is shown as increased respiratory rate, use of accessory muscles and grunting
Inhalational chemical injury	A history of having inhaled a potentially hazardous chemical. Some chemicals may leave specific signs while others may not. The nature of the hazard may not be immediately apparent
Inhalational injury	A history of being confined in a smoke filled space is the most reliable indicator of smoke inhalation. Carbon deposits around the mouth and nose and hoarse voice may be present. History is also the most reliable way of diagnosing inhalation of chemicals – there will not necessarily be any signs
Insecure airway	Patients who cannot continually maintain their own airway have an insecure airway
Known immunosuppression	Any patient on immunosuppressive drugs (including long term steroids) or who is HIV positive
Lethality	The potential of the substance taken to cause illness or death. Advice from a Poisons Centre may be required to establish this. If in doubt assume a high risk
Local infection	Local infection usually manifests as inflammation (pain, swelling and redness) confined to a particular site or area, with or without a collection of pus
Local inflammation	Local inflammation will involve pain, swelling and redness confined to a particular site or area
Low PEFR	This is a PEFR of 50% or less of best or predicted PEFR
Low SaO_2	This is a saturation of <95% on air
Marked distress	Patients who are markedly physically or emotionally upset fulfil this criterion
Moderate itch	An itch that is bearable but intense
Moderate lethality	Lethality is the potential of the substance taken to cause serious illness or death. Advice from a Poisons Centre may be required to establish the level of risk to the patient
Moderate lethality envenomation	Lethality is the potential of the envenomation to cause harm. Local knowledge may allow identification of the venomous creature, but advice may be required

Moderate pain	Pain that is bearable but intense. See the chapter on pain assessment
Moderate risk of (further) harm to others	The presence of a potential risk of harm to others can be judged by looking at posture (tense and clenched), speech patterns (loud and using threatening words) and motor behaviour (restless, pacing). Moderate risk should be assumed if there is any indication of potential harm to others
Moderate risk of (further) self-harm	An initial view of the risk of self-harm can be formed by considering the patients' behaviour. Patients without a significant history of self-harm, who are not actively trying to harm themselves, who are not actively trying to leave with the intent of harming themselves, but who profess the desire to harm themselves are at moderate risk
New neurological deficit	Any loss of neurological function including altered or lost sensation, weakness of the limbs (either transiently or permanently) and alterations in bladder or bowel function
No improvement with own asthma medications	This history should be available from the patient. A failure to improve with bronchodilator therapy given by the GP or paramedic is equally significant
Non-blanching rash	A rash that does not blanch (go white) when pressure is applied to it. Often tested using a glass tumbler to apply pressure as any colour change can be observed through the bottom of the tumbler
Normal menstruation	Menstrual blood loss and pain occurring on the expected date for the expected length of time
Not distractible	Children who are distressed by pain or other things who cannot be distracted by conversation or play fulfil this criterion
Not feeding	Children who will not take any solid or liquid (as appropriate) by mouth. Children who will take the food but always vomit afterwards may also fulfil this criterion
Not passing urine	Failure to produce and pass urine. This may be difficult to judge in children (and the elderly) and reference to the number of nappies or pads used may be useful
Oedema of the tongue	Swelling of the tongue of any degree

Open fracture	All wounds in the vicinity of a fracture should be regarded with suspicion. If there is any possibility of communication between the wound and the fracture then the fracture should be assumed to be open
Pain on joint movement	This can be pain on either active (patient) movement or passive (examiner) movement
Pain radiating to the back	Pain that is also felt in the back either intermittently or constantly
Passing fresh or altered blood PR	In active massive GI bleeding dark red blood will be passed PR. As GI transit time increases this becomes darker, eventually becoming melaena
PEFR <33% predicted	The peak expiratory flow rate predicted after consideration of the age and sex of the patient. Some patients may know their 'best' PEFR and this may be used. If the ratio of measured to predicted is less than 33% then this criterion is fulfilled
PEFR <50% predicted	The peak expiratory flow rate predicted after consideration of the age and sex of the patient. Some patients may know their 'best' PEFR and this may be used. If the ratio of measured to predicted is less than 50% then this criterion is fulfilled
Penetrating eye injury	A recent physically traumatic event involving penetration of the globe
Penetrating trauma	A recent physically traumatic event which involves discrete penetration of any body area by a knife, bullet or other object
Persistent vomiting	Vomiting that is continuous or that occurs without any respite between episodes
Pleuritic pain	A sharp, localised pain in the chest that worsens on breathing, coughing or sneezing
Possibly pregnant	Any woman whose normal menstruation has failed to occur is possibly pregnant. Furthermore any woman of childbearing age who is having unprotected sex should be considered to be potentially pregnant
Presenting foetal parts	Crowning or presentation of any other foetal part in the vagina
Priapism	Sustained penile erection
Prolapsed umbilical cord	Prolapse of any part of the umbilical cord through the cervix

Prolonged or uninterrupted crying	A child who has cried continuously for 2 hours or more fulfils this criterion
Pulse rate abnormal	If the capillary refill time cannot be measured then major incident casualties whose pulse is raised over 120 beats per minute are categorised RED
Purpura	A rash on any part of the body that is caused by small haemorrhages under the skin. A purpuric rash does not blanch (go white) when pressure is applied to it
PV blood loss	Any loss of blood per vaginum
PV blood loss and more than 20 weeks pregnant	Any loss of blood per vaginum in a woman known to be beyond the 20th week of pregnancy
Rapid onset	Onset within the preceding 12 hours
Recent hearing loss	Loss of hearing in one or both ears within the previous week
Recent injury	An injury occurring within the last week is said to be recent
Recent mild itch	Any itch that has occurred in the past 7 days
Recent mild pain	Any pain that has occurred within the past 7 days
Recent problem	A problem arising in the last week is said to be recent
Recent reduced visual acuity	Any reduction in corrected visual acuity within the past 7 days
Recent signs of mild pain	Young children and babies in pain cannot complain. They will usually cry occasionally and may act atypically
Redcurrant stool	A dark red stool classically seen in intersussception. Absence of this type of stool does not rule out the diagnosis
Red eye	Any redness to the eye. A red eye may be painful or painless and may be complete or partial
Respiratory rate	Major incident casualties whose respiratory rate is abnormal either by being too high (over 29) or too low (less than 10) are categorised as RED
Responds to pain	Response to a painful stimulus. Standard peripheral stimuli should be used – a pencil or pen is used to apply pressure to the finger nail bed. This stimulus should not be applied to the toes since a spinal reflex may cause flexion even in brain death. Supraorbital ridge pressure should not be used since reflex grimacing may occur

Responds to voice	Response to a vocal stimulus. It is not necessary to shout the patients' name. Children may fail to respond because they are afraid
Retention of urine	Inability to pass urine per urethra associated with an enlarged bladder. This condition is usually very painful unless there is altered sensation
Risk of continued contamination	If chemical exposure is likely to continue (usually due to lack of adequate decontamination) then this discriminator applies. Risks to health care workers must not be forgotten if this situation occurs
Risk of harm to others	The potential of the patient to actively attempt to harm others. This may be assessed by considering the state of mind, body posture and behaviour. If in doubt assume a high risk
Risk of self-harm	The potential of the patient to actively attempt further self-harm. If in doubt assume a high risk
Scalp haematoma	A raised bruised area to the scalp (bruises below the hair line at the front are to the forehead)
Scrotal cellulitis	Redness and swelling around the scrotum
Scrotal gangrene	Dead blackened skin around the scrotum and groin. Early gangrene may not be black but may appear like a full thickness burn with or without flaking
Scrotal trauma	Any recent physically traumatic event involving the scrotum
Severe itch	An itch that is unbearable
Severe pain	Pain that is unbearable – often described as the worst ever. See the chapter on pain assessment
Shock	Shock is inadequate delivery of oxygen to the tissues. The classical signs include sweating, pallor, tachycardia, hypotension and reduced conscious level
Shoulder tip pain	Pain felt in the tip of the shoulder. This often indicates diaphragmatic irritation
Significant cardiac history	A known recurrent dysrhythmia which has life-threatening effects is significant as is a known cardiac condition that may deteriorate rapidly
Significant haematological history	A patient with a haematological disorder that is known to deteriorate rapidly
Significant history of allergy	A known sensitivity with severe reaction (e.g. to nuts or bee sting) is significant

Significant history of GI bleed	Any history of massive GI bleeding or of any GI bleed associated with oesophageal varices
Significant mechanism of injury	Penetrating injuries (stab or gunshot) and injuries with high energy transfer such as falls from heights and high speed road traffic accidents (speed >40 mph) are significant especially if there has been ejection from the vehicle, death(s) of other victim(s) of the accident or marked deformation of the vehicle
Significant medical history	Any pre-existing medical condition requiring continual medication or other care
Significant psychiatric history	A history of a major psychiatric illness or event
Significant respiratory history	A history of previous life threatening episodes of a respiratory condition (e.g. COPD) is significant as is brittle asthma
Signs of dehydration	These include dry tongue, sunken eyes, increased skin turgor and, in small babies, a sunken anterior fontanelle. Usually associated with a low urine output
Signs of meningism	Classically a stiff neck together with headache and photophobia
Signs of moderate pain	Young children and babies in moderate pain cannot complain. They will usually cry intermittently and are often intermittently consolable
Signs of severe pain	Young children and babies in severe pain cannot complain. They will usually cry out continuously and inconsolably and be tachycardic. They may well exhibit signs such as pallor and sweating
Smoke inhalation	Smoke inhalation should be assumed if the patient has been confined in a smoke filled space. Physical signs such as oral or nasal soot are less reliable but significant if present
Special risk of infection	Known exposure to a dangerous pathogen, or travel to an area with an identified, current serious infectious risk
Stridor	This may be an inspiratory or expiratory noise, or both. Stridor is heard best on breathing with the mouth open
Subcutaneous gas	Gas under the skin can be detected by feeling for a 'crackling' on touch. There may be gas bubbles and a line of demarcation

Swelling	An abnormal increase in size
Temporal scalp tenderness	Tenderness on palpation over the temporal area (especially over the artery)
Testicular pain	Pain in the testicles
Threatening to others	Patients with threatening posture (tense and clenched), speech patterns (loud and using threatening words) and motor behaviour (restless, pacing)
TRTS	Triage revised trauma score: this is calculated using the coded respiratory rate (0–4), the systolic blood pressure (0–4) and the Glasgow Coma Scale score (0–4) to give a score from 0 to 12. This scoring system is shown on most triage labels
Unable to feed	This is usually reported by the parents. Children who will not take any solid or liquid (as appropriate) by mouth
Unable to talk in sentences	Patients who are so breathless that they cannot complete relatively short sentences in one breath
Unable to walk	It is important to try and distinguish between patients who have pain and difficulty walking and those who *cannot* walk. Only the latter can be said to be unable to walk
Uncontrollable major haemorrhage	A haemorrhage that is not rapidly controlled by the application of sustained direct pressure and in which blood continues to flow heavily or soak through large dressings quickly
Uncontrollable minor haemorrhage	A haemorrhage that is not rapidly controlled by the application of sustained direct pressure and in which blood continues to flow slightly or ooze
Unresponsive	Patients who fail to respond to either verbal or painful stimuli are unresponsive
Unresponsive child	A child who fails to respond to either verbal or painful stimuli is unresponsive
Vaginal trauma	Any history or other evidence of direct trauma to the vagina fulfils this criterion
Vascular compromise	There will be a combination of pallor, coldness, altered sensation and pain with or without absent pulses distal to the injury
Vertigo	An acute feeling of spinning or dizziness, possibly accompanied by nausea and vomiting

Very hot adult	If the skin feels very hot the patient is clinically said to be very hot. The temperature should be taken as soon as possible – a temperature >41°C is very hot
Very low PEFR	This is a PEFR of 33% or less of best or predicted PEFR
Very low SaO$_2$	This is a saturation <95% on O$_2$ therapy or <90% on air
Visible abdominal mass	A mass in the abdomen that is visible to the naked eye
Vomiting	Any emesis fulfils this criterion
Vomiting blood	Vomited blood may be fresh (bright or dark red) or coffee ground in appearance
Walking	In a major incident any patient who can walk fulfils this criterion
Warmth	If the skin feels warm the patient is clinically said to be warm. The temperature should be taken as soon as possible – a temperature >37.5°C is warm
Wheeze	This can be audible wheeze or a feeling of wheeze. Very severe airway obstruction is silent (no air can move)
Widespread rash or blistering	Any discharging or blistering eruption covering more than 10% body surface area
Wound contamination	A wound that contains extrinsic material of any description is said to be contaminated

Index